THE HERBAL APPRENTICE
AND OTHER STORIES

THE HERBAL APPRENTICE AND OTHER STORIES
Tales from a Plant Medicine Practitioner

Andrew Chevallier

AEON

First published in 2026 by
Aeon Books

British Library Cataloguing in Publication Data

A C.I.P. for this book is available from the British Library

ISBN-13: 978-1-80152-100-0

Typeset by Medlar Publishing Solutions Pvt Ltd, India

www.aeonbooks.co.uk

CONTENTS

FOREWORD

by Anne McIntyre

What a wonderfully engaging, entertaining, and at the same time educational collection of stories. Some of the tales really made me smile, and they will resonate with many readers, not only those familiar with the herbal world. I loved the descriptions of the arduous training, days and weeks studying at the School of Herbal Medicine, student clinics and terrifying final exams ... they brought back memories that hadn't come to mind for decades!

How unusual it is to read a book about herbs and herbal practice through stories of real life: exchanges between a herbalist and his patients, meetings with friends, herbs walks, hospital visits, hiking in Wales searching for herbs. And what a privilege it is to be allowed glimpses of the musings and hindsight about these herbal ventures, a life behind the practitioner. I doubt that many herbalists would be so brave and honest to describe not only their successes, but also the things they would not do again! Bringing herbal practice to life in this way is such a great way for the reader to learn about herbs and what it means to be a practitioner. I sense that Andrew loves Valerian root as it comes up several times in his stories, and I'm reminded to use Angelica root more in my practice.

Naturally my curiosity has got the better of me and I'm longing to know how much of each story is true and how much is fiction. Was Andrew really inspired to start training after searching for treatment of a debilitating illness? Did he really work in a printshop and live in Kent? Was he really the teenage author of a two thousand word essay on existentialism?

In the end what really comes across for me is the insight, patience, and compassion to be found within these stories. They speak of a herbalist going beyond the call of duty for patients and friends, of wise and often difficult decisions, and challenges much like those that we inevitably meet ourselves in practice from time to time.

Fittingly the book ends on a philosophical note with a moving tale about the transformational power of intense hardship in life, as he describes a boy's persecution at school and its effects, reflected perhaps in the last story in the book, about a chrysalis and emerging butterfly in Colombia … what a brilliant way to end! Thank you, Andrew!

Anne McIntyre FNIMH, MAPA, MCPP

What started out as an idea for a book for students called *The Herbal Apprentice* morphed over time into this little book of short stories. I found that after years of writing practical books on herbal medicine, I had come to the end of that road. I wanted the freedom to write from experience, to give some flavour of what it takes to train and practise as a medical herbalist and reveal in passing what a rich, complex world it is.

As the project developed, the attraction of writing short stories took over. I was not going to be rigidly bound by subject matter—I would follow a meandering path, if that seemed the best course to take. Of the twenty-three stories in this book, most do revolve around herbal medicine in one way or another, but there are some that have gone their own way and focus on chance meetings, insignificant moments or a day's outing.

It goes without saying that the characters who live within these short stores are fictional and have no life beyond these pages. I have tried, however, to retain the emotional and intellectual truth that can sometimes be found, often in unexpected ways, to underlie real-life encounters and events.

Lastly, and to my surprise, it seems to me that some of the stories contain a quiet, playful humour. It's definitely understated, but there's a chance that it might bring the occasional smile to your face.

THE HERBAL APPRENTICE

Twenty-Seven

I was not feeling well but there was nothing to be done about it. I took my two-year-old son Euan round to friends for the night, as arranged, and went on to the printshop to do my last shift, before setting off for Scotland and my parents the following day. I knew I was pushing it but I needed the night's wages to pay for the train tickets.

By the time we reached Euston and had found our way to the Inverness train, I was worse—throbbing head, sore throat and aching muscles. It was too late to turn back and, in any case, Vicki was at an ecology conference in Turin and wasn't back till the end of the week. At my parents, I could rest and my mother would be happy to look after Euan.

Euan behaved as never before on that six-hour train journey—he didn't run off down the corridor, he didn't cry, he ate his food without splurging and spitting it out. He knew things weren't right and didn't want to make them worse. He sat calmly on my lap, looking out of the window or playing on the table with his toys, no protest, no complaints.

Arriving at Stirling, I was feverish and weak, struggling to carry my rucksack, while at the same time shepherding Euan off the train. Thankfully, my parents were there waiting and we climbed into the car.

I saw my mother's shocked look as she saw how ill I was, and she took over. All I was good for was bed.

Day after day in bed and I wasn't sure I was going to get better. The doctor prescribed antibiotics but I knew I had a viral infection. It wasn't bacterial, so I didn't take them. I'd never liked taking tablets, not even paracetamol or aspirin. During that first week, when I still had a fever the only things that made a difference were fresh garlic, strong chamomile tea and glasses of tonic water—*not* all at the same time. The fever, aches and pains and headache all eased a little after taking them, symptoms slowly returning as their effects wore off.

It was a warm sunny end to September, and while I remained in bed with the curtains drawn, my mother took Euan off for walks and to play by a local stream. Vicki arrived several days later, deeply worried. It was very good to see her but I had almost no energy to talk or share emotion with her, and after just a few minutes' talking, I had to turn over and rest. We agreed she would go back to London with Euan and I would follow, when I was up to it.

Recovery was painfully slow. I carried on with the chamomile and garlic. Everything was done in small doses—some music on the radio, a few paragraphs of a book, just looking at the trees out of the window. After three weeks, I got up and ate lunch at the table. Another week and my first foray into the outside world for a month. We drove to a local loch and I stayed in the car while my parents took the dogs off for a walk. I clambered unsteadily out of the car, looking at the shimmering water and surrounding hills, and breathing in the icy air. When the dogs came bounding back, I went to pick up a stick to throw for them—but I had no strength to pick it up, let alone throw it.

As I got slowly better, I saw that life would not be the same when I got back to London, and I appreciated the quiet time spent with my mother and father, their care and support. We had good conversations, played Scrabble in the evenings, avoided politics, and felt closer to each other than we had for many years.

Finally, the day came when I caught the train back home. It was a great release but daunting. I was quite out of practice at being in the midst of crowds and people all about—the rush and crush of trains and stations. My stamina ran out long before I reached Euston. I had to pause every so often in the Underground to get my strength back and then, up the steps to arrive in fading daylight at Highbury Corner, snarled up as usual with rush-hour traffic, the air thick with fumes.

In through the front door and at last I was home, being hugged and kissed by Vicki and Euan. I sat down at the kitchen table, shaking with exhaustion, and saw the "Welcome Home, Tom" card that the two of them had made. Vicki had cooked a vegetable moussaka, one of my favourite meals. It was a joy to be back but I was overwhelmed and so tired I could not eat—after a few mouthfuls I had to apologise and, dismayed, crawled my way upstairs to bed.

The days passed slowly. Stuck on a plateau, I was not recovering. Quickly fatigued, I snapped at Euan—something that had rarely happened before—and struggled to cope with looking after him two days a week. I slept twelve hours at a time and it took days to feel half well again. It was not much better with Vicki—she wanted to go out when we could find a babysitter, to the cinema, to friends, to see a band and dance in the local club or community centre. She was trying to be patient with me but I could see the patience wearing thin, and she began to visit friends in the evening, leaving me with Euan once he'd gone to sleep.

I had given up smoking and was trying to eat better. It was bad enough being flat and having no energy, I thought, but resisting the urge to smoke after a meal crowned it all. I had no idea what to do. There was no way I could work at the printshop and I had lost much of my freelance work—I couldn't meet the deadlines required. I was still managing to write the odd article and had a class teaching Creative Writing, though this was the other side of London and just two hours a week.

Money issues were ever present. I had come through being acutely ill believing that I would bounce back to good health, but now, weak and unwell, anxious and low-spirited, I felt oppressed, as if my old life and all its certainties were being stripped away one by one.

I told myself that this was the darkest hour and that dawn was around the corner, but it didn't feel like that. I was stuck in a pit and didn't have the strength to climb out. Perhaps, it's only when we are vulnerable that we truly recognise how much we depend on others. The rest of the time, we assert and pretend to independence, telling ourselves that we can survive perfectly well on our own. There's an old saying that if you're all tied up—tightly knotted ropes round wrists and ankles—you need somebody else to come and release you. My pride, like my body, had taken a battering but it meant that I was ready to accept help whenever it was offered.

Vicki invited an old friend from her schooldays round for supper one evening. Sandra had just qualified as an osteopath, and after we'd eaten, she took me aside and said that Vicki was really worried about me, and that she, Sandra, could see that I was struggling and still unwell. We talked about my exhaustion, fuzzy head and other symptoms, and she suggested I see her acupuncturist, Lian Xing, as well as a medical herbalist she knew in north London. Both would help me on the path back to good health.

With her sensitive questioning and advice, Sandra renewed faith that I could get well again. What is more important, I asked myself, than the belief that you *will* get better, that a new chapter, new horizons, lie ahead? The next day Sandra phoned Lian Xing and made an appointment for me. Later, she phoned me with the details of the appointment and told me it was a birthday present. Twenty-seven that week, I could not have asked for a more thoughtful gift.

That night, in the early hours, I woke to find myself sobbing uncontrollably into the pillow, pain and grief bursting forth in breathless moans that seemed to claw up from the depths and force their way out through my throat and mouth. Vicki held me tight and tried to comfort me but for a while I was far away and inconsolable, lost in suffering and the inarticulate world of emotional pain. In the morning, I woke drained but aware of a sense of release, of relief, as if I had been cleansed in some way, and become lighter, cleaner, sharper. Determined to make the most of this, I called Emily Marshall, the medical herbalist and doctor that Sandra had recommended, and made an initial appointment for an hour the following week.

Needles

Lian Xing ushered me into the room and pointed to the chair. She was Chinese and though small in stature her movements betrayed a deep inner discipline and strength. Her dark brown eyes examined me intensely through wisps of black hair, and I felt as if I was being put under a microscope. She spent a long time studying my face and then tongue, took both pulses, made some clucking noises and directed me, in not very good English, to lie down on the couch.

Acupuncture was new to me. I lay down in the semi-dark and waited for the needles. It was a strange sensation, the needles barely hurt, except when she came back to twist them. After a while, she moved around, holding a burning stick of dried mugwort in her hand, pointing its glowing tip to warm specific points on my body. The room began to fill with acrid-smelling smoke. When she'd finished, she stubbed out the stick and went back to the office, her silence proving more unsettling than the treatment. I lay there for a long time, shooting and tingling feelings in my body, until she returned and swiftly removed the needles. Again, not a word.

Sitting back in the consulting room, she finished writing her notes and then, looking up directly at me, said, almost with a measure of distaste, "You, Tom, are like the man who is permanently overdrawn at the bank—you cannot spend any money, any energy, till you have healthy credit balance!"

My throat tightened, I couldn't swallow—no one had ever spoken to me before with such shocking accuracy. She was right, she had just held up a mirror and forced me to confront exactly how I was. I could only admire her perceptiveness and economy. The acupuncture undoubtedly helped, but her words were delivered as precisely as the needles. They struck home and could be neither ignored nor forgotten.

I *was* depleted, demoralised, low in energy, overdrawn at the bank—both metaphorically and literally. Instead of slowly rebuilding and moving forwards, saving and conserving the little energy I had to spare, I was still recklessly spending it, trying to live the life I had before. As if those youthful, seemingly inexhaustible, reserves of energy were still there to be drawn on. Deep within, I was mourning that loss and unwilling to learn a new way of being, one that did not make excess demands and thrust my body back into deficit each time.

"Go to Tai Chi class", continued Lian Xing, "at least once a week. This will strengthen *chi*. And you are eating wrong food. You must only eat warm, cooked food, not cold or fried."

A few days later I started a Tai Chi class in central London—something I have continued with—but it was Lian Xing's words that I kept returning to. I knew now that only by rebuilding my stamina and vitality and by acquiring the self-discipline to minimise energy use, would I get well again.

Angelica root

Encouraged by Sandra, I borrowed books on herbal medicine from the library and began to discover a world I knew little about. As a child, on country walks with my father, I'd learnt the names of wildflowers from the commonest, such as dandelion, elder and foxglove, through to rarer plants such as betony, dodder and woody nightshade. I loved them for their beauty and form and colour. I'd never thought about them as medicines, as having curative powers, but now I was determined to learn more. If herbal medicine could help me to recover and be well that would be good, but I also wanted to help Euan and Vicki to stay well and to have natural treatments at hand should any of us fall ill in the future.

I got off the bus in Crouch End and, taking care to conserve my energy, walked slowly up the hill to the tree-lined street where Emily Marshall practised. Large Edwardian houses set in good-sized gardens bordered the road, and it didn't take long to find the right house, crocuses, hellebore and witchhazel all in flower, as I walked up the path to the Clinic at the side entrance to the house. The receptionist, Fi, let me in and apologised that Dr Marshall was running ten minutes late.

Sitting in the waiting area, I watched Fi through a hatch, as she returned to dispensing in the pharmacy, taking one brown glass bottle after another off the shelves, pulling out the stopper, measuring carefully and then pouring the contents into the bottle being dispensed. There were more than a hundred bottles of tincture, arranged like books along the shelves, with many more large jars with dried herbs and smaller containers of creams, oils and tablets. An aromatic but not entirely pleasant smell drifted through the hatch.

It was a whole new world to me. There was something enticing yet familiar about it, that these plants had been grown, harvested, dried and brought from across the world to this corner of London, to be used as medicines and to heal. How long would it take to learn to be able to use them all safely and effectively, I wondered.

Looking around the reception area there were pot plants, colourful posters of medicinal plants and their uses on the wall, a filing cabinet and hanging above the reception desk a small plaque. I went over to look at it more closely and was astonished to find a Coat of Arms that had an ancient Egyptian goddess to one side and a native American in a loincloth and long feather headdress to the other. Between them was the heraldic shield of the National Institute of Medical Herbalists, founded, so the plaque said, in 1864, bearing three white roses and twigs of what looked like rosemary.

I was absorbed in looking at this when Emily Marshall came out of the consulting room, and walked over and introduced herself. She was about 50, with longish dark greying hair, questioning blue eyes, and a sharply intelligent face. She was dressed professionally and wore a pearl necklace behind a pale cream blouse. I could see she was sizing me up as she walked towards me and didn't think much of my black leather jacket and spiky hair. "It's Tom, isn't it," she said with a practised smile, as we shook hands, and then looking up at the Coat of Arms, "It's not quite what you'd expect, is it!"

There was a large oak desk to one side of the consulting room, an examination couch along the wall on the other side, and van Gogh and Degas prints on the wall. We sat down in the middle on semi-comfy chairs set at roughly 90° to each other. Giving me time to settle, Emily said, "So what brings you here, what can I do for you?" her head tilted attentively to one side.

After preparing for this moment for so long and already feeling mentally tired, my words came out jumbled, all at one and the same time, as I began to tell her my symptoms, how exhausted I was, how low I felt and how I'd come to be ill.

"Perhaps, you can tell me how you are feeling right now—are you in pain? What is the most important problem?" she prompted.

I took a deep breath in and began again. I'd been chronically exhausted for months, it felt as if a cloud was hanging over me all the time. I never woke refreshed after a night's sleep, I was irritable and anxious in a way I had never been before, I often had a sore throat and fuzzy headache, it was hard to concentrate … she listened closely and let me talk away, every so often interrupting to reassure or clarify a point.

"How did all these symptoms come about?" Emily asked, and I told her about working the shift in the printshop, the journey to Scotland, and the weeks spent in bed at my parents'. She asked many more questions, some predictable, some unexpected, such as whether I tended to get too hot or too cold, and I answered as best I could.

She took my pulse and blood pressure, looked at my mouth and into my throat and said she wanted to examine my abdomen. I lay down on the couch and she carefully pressed and palpated all around my stomach area, asking if there was pain or discomfort. On the right side, as she pushed, I felt twinges of pain and nausea. "I think your liver may be enlarged and your gallbladder somewhat inflamed," she said, "but don't worry, this should be something that can be sorted out quickly."

Back in our chairs, she took a while to collect her thoughts and then began to give me her assessment. "It's very likely that what you've had is glandular fever, although you're old to get it at 27. Low energy and a very slow recovery often occur with glandular fever. The virus attacks the glandular system, including the liver, and leaves the immune system weakened. I am confident that with the right treatment you will get better, but it will take time. If your recovery is like other patients I've treated with glandular fever, it will be a case of 'three steps forward and two steps back'—you need to be patient and, as far as possible, not exhaust yourself." All this she said matter-of-factly, but with an undertone of warmth and concern that was deeply reassuring.

Next, she gave me a diet sheet, with strict instructions to avoid most fats and oils, including dairy produce, all processed foods, poor-quality meat and alcohol. I should eat food as close to its natural state as possible. She suggested some supplements and recommended chamomile, ginger and thyme as infusions.

I waited as she worked out my prescription, feeling encouraged and more positive than I had felt for a long time—some of the cloud had lifted!

"I'm going to give you a simple prescription to start with and see how you get on with it. I'd like to see you again in two weeks' time. How you respond will help me refine the prescription, so that it is targeted more precisely. The herbs I'm giving you now are: blue flag, calendula, dandelion root, echinacea, golden seal and thyme."

She gave a brief explanation of why she had selected each herb: "dandelion has been shown in clinical studies to promote healthy liver function, golden seal is thought to be a specific for glandular fever" … and then gave me clear instructions on how to take the tincture.

"You should begin to see an improvement within a week or so," she said, looking me directly in the eyes, "but the rule is you that can only spend 50% of this gain, the other 50% you have to save. It's very easy to get carried away. If you suddenly find you have energy to spare, the temptation is to start doing too much and exhaust yourself. That way the treatment won't work." I nodded in agreement, laughing within—she was saying what Lian Xing had said before, though in a less severe way.

The hour was over. We went out into reception and Emily gave Fi the prescription to dispense. I thanked Emily for her help and sat down again, watching through the hatch as Fi made up my herbal prescription.

Back outside it was raining but as I walked back down the hill to Crouch End, the tincture bottle in my jacket pocket, my step was lighter and my heart more at ease than it had been for weeks.

The tincture tasted terrible but I took it the three times a day before each meal. Euan watched me drinking it and made a show of going "Phoo" every time he smelt it, then ran off, with a flash of his cheeky smile. The upbeat mood lasted for about three days and then fell away, leaving me staring once again into a gloomy, all too familiar world. After a week there was no sign of more energy but I was sleeping better and my head was clearer. Just before the two weeks were up, Vicki confided in me that she thought I was getting less tired—it wasn't obvious, but she could see it in the way I was approaching tasks in a more methodical, organised way. I hoped she was right.

I reported all this back to Emily, when I saw her at the follow-up appointment. She questioned me closely, took my pulse and said she was pleased with my progress—my skin tone and the colour of my face had improved, my pulse was stronger and I was sleeping better. It was often the case in chronic health conditions that change was almost imperceptible to begin with. I wanted to believe her but was sceptical.

She smiled and said, "You haven't mentioned the sore throat—has that been a problem over the last two weeks?" She'd caught me by surprise, no, I hadn't had a sore throat and I had to admit that I hadn't noticed that it had gone.

"I'm going to make a minor change to your prescription," Emily said. "I'm taking out blue flag and replacing it with angelica root. This is a warming, tonic, mildly bitter herb that should help you to give you better stamina and to be less tired."

I started taking the new prescription as soon as I got home—it tasted almost pleasant in comparison with the first one. As I sipped the tincture, I thought of the candied angelica stems that my mother had used to decorate her cakes, when I was a child. After two days, I felt warmer and was less breathless when walking. A few days later and I was feeling better than at any time since getting ill. I woke earlier in the morning, most often feeling clear-headed and was able to get out of bed straight away.

Simple everyday tasks started to get easier and didn't leave me drained. I was amazed that as my energy began to return, so my mood lightened and rather than a forced smile, I found myself smiling and laughing for no good reason. I took Euan to the park—it had been too far for me to go before—pushed him on the swings and roundabouts and managed to get back home without feeling exhausted. Vicki and I went out for a meal together—our first for over four months.

At our next appointment, Emily expressed delight at hearing how much I had improved. Provided I didn't exhaust myself, she told me, the improvement should continue until I was fully well again. I had to be careful and pace myself and must not to try to run before I could walk.

Could I begin to think about working full-time again, I asked? She looked thoughtful and said that in six to eight weeks' time and, provided I eased myself slowly back into work, it should be perfectly possible. As she said this, I could feel tears welling up in my eyes—I was going to get my life back—and I told her how much I appreciated her help. Emily said I needed to continue with the tincture, supplements and diet for at least another three months.

As we walked out to reception, I asked if there was a course on herbal medicine she could recommend—I was really interested in what medicinal plants could do and wanted to learn more. She stopped, appraising me in a quite different way, a softer tone to her voice, "Yes, you should contact the School of Herbal Medicine in Tunbridge Wells. They offer a one-year self-help course and a four-year course leading to professional practice as a member of the National Institute of Medical Herbalists. I'm sure they will be able to help you." I wrote down the details and, having waited to collect my tincture, went back down the street, almost skipping.

The Herbal Apprentice

We headed out on the Westway and onto the M4, a sense of excitement building as we left the city behind, aiming for Wales and the Brecon Beacons, and a long weekend away. After two hours we stopped for coffee at the services by the Severn Bridge and sitting next to the window looked out over the estuary and its coursing waters far below.

"It's got the second largest tidal range in the world," said Mike, scanning the horizon, but I was looking down at the swirling water, thinking that it was a year since I'd gone to Scotland with Euan and become so ill. What a year! I'd doubted that I would ever be well again, and now here I was in a full-time job and off to hike in the hills.

"You're far away," Mike said, interrupting my thoughts and finishing his coffee. "You've got to live in the moment, you know." I smiled at him and pulled a face—he was a good friend and fun to be with, but he could be brusque at times.

We crossed the bridge into Wales and stopped at a supermarket in Abergavenny. Leaving the main road, my little Fiat took the twisting corners and gradients of the lanes with ease, as we drew close to the cottage we'd rented in Capel-y-ffin. I hadn't been on a serious hike since getting ill, and in the back of my mind lingered the fear that it might be too much. Mike understood that we needed to take it slowly to begin with, but I knew he was champing to get some 'miles in'. We'd chosen the cottage because it was not too far from Hay-on-Wye, and if it rained non-stop, or I needed to rest, we could spend hours browsing in the second-hand bookshops and hanging out in cafés.

We unpacked, had a late lunch, and got out the Ordnance Survey map. "Something gentle to break us in?" Mike intoned, pointing out a circular route of about 5 miles with his finger.

"As long as there aren't too many steep climbs, and don't expect me to keep up with you, if you start yomping away."

"It's just straight up the hillside, along the moorland top for about two miles, then down and back along the road. It should be easy." I knew from experience what 'easy' meant for Mike, so wasn't totally reassured.

It had rained a lot and the ground was wet and sodden, which made it slippery at times. I quickly got out of breath, legs complaining at the effort, but as we climbed up the scarp out of the valley the sun came out and we began to see over the surrounding hills. Mike raced on ahead, and when I reached the top, I found him sitting on a rock looking out at the heather and bracken-covered hills that stretched away into the distance.

I sat down and ate some oatcakes. Once rested, we set off, striding across the springy turf, following the path as it snaked round the crest of the hill and then ran gently uphill towards the next peak. After half an hour walking along the top, I began to ease into a comfortable, regular stride in time with Mike's. Slowly, that feeling that comes when out walking in the wild—the tramp of the boots, the silence and sense of space, the breeze, the birdsong, the bees on the heather—crept up on me, and I realised I *was* alive and full of energy, that the illness was now behind me, and that I was truly well again. It was a wonderful moment.

A little further on, we found the path for the descent back down to the road, and once we'd worked our way through the bracken, I just ran, hopping, skipping, leaving Mike far behind, down through the fields towards the road, skirting the thistles and hummocks, and reaching the road panting but grinning, a fierce joy in my heart.

The cottage was damp and we lit the coal fire in the rather pokey living room, then sat around it talking and reminiscing—we hadn't seen each other for months. Mike was a furniture designer and restorer. I knew he'd been struggling to make his way but now, as he told me that he was getting busier with more one-off commissions, I could see that he was more self-assured. He was leasing a large studio/workshop near Portobello Road, where he would be able to see clients and exhibit his furniture. He was going to live there too, he explained—he and Paula had finally split up, though they remained good friends. I wasn't going to hold my breath on that, I said to myself—their relationship had been on and off so many times over the years that I'd lost count.

Mike sensed my thinking and changed the subject, asking about my job at the housing association. It was fine, a good place to work, I told him. I liked the people and the work, and could leave early to pick up Euan from the nursery, but long term it wasn't what I wanted. Mike looked puzzled and I told him the secret—I'd signed up on the distance learning course at the School of Herbal Medicine and was aiming to qualify and practise as a medical herbalist. I had my first piece of home-work to do over the weekend.

It would be tough, very tough—the course was four years with week-long sessions at the School in Tunbridge Wells and clinical training on top, and all this while working full-time—but Vicki and I had talked it over and she was keen to support me, despite it meaning that I would have much less time to look after Euan. He was at nursery four days a week now, so it was less of a problem.

* * *

The next morning, we woke to rain beating on the roof, the hills covered in cloud. Hoping that the weather would improve, we took our time over breakfast, but it grew darker and carried on raining. A day for chilling out in bookshops, we realised, and made for Hay.

There are so many second-hand bookshops in Hay-on-Wye that you could spend weeks trawling through them. After browsing four shops and buying two books, one on woodworking and one an art book on Magritte, Mike decided he'd had enough and was going to sit in a café and read and maybe buy the paper.

Walking on down the street I found myself outside a former cinema, now a vast second-hand bookshop. I went in, gasping at its scale—the size of a public library, there were books on shelves everywhere, all indexed by subject matter. I lost track of time scouting along the aisles looking for herbal and medical books. There weren't that many but I found and bought three: an illustrated anatomy textbook, *Welsh Herbal*

Medicine (Abercastle, 1978) by David Hoffmann, and—I couldn't resist it—*Coffin's Botanical Medicine* (London, 1866). Just the title evoked Dickens and Victorian London, though surprisingly, Dr Coffin was an American.

I met up with Mike and we had lunch. The rain had eased off and we drove back up into the hills for another walk. The ground was so sodden and boggy, we decided to stick to lanes and tracks that skirted the forest plantations.

Back in the house, I put tired feet up on a stool and told Mike I was going to do a couple of hours' homework. He gave me a pitying look but said, not to worry, he'd do the supper.

The first project was a sample Herbarium—I had to choose a common native medicinal plant, such as dandelion or nettle, and:

A) Write a short summary of the plant's botany, constituents and medicinal actions and indications.
B) Find a healthy plant in flower, collect it with as much of the roots as possible, carefully press it and, when dry, mount it. Then list and identify its key botanical features.

The project had to be handed in at the first week-long session at the School, so I had three weeks to complete it. I'd chosen yarrow. I'd always loved its tough yet delicate beauty, feathery leaves and clusters of off-white or pinkish flowers set on a terminal head. It was in flower everywhere, including the garden surrounding the cottage. I was going to dig up one of the plants just before we left, put it in a moistened plastic bag and press it as soon as I got home.

I'd brought a flora with me but opted to read the chapters on yarrow in my new books first. From *Welsh Herbal Medicine*, I learnt that yarrow was a standard treatment for flus and colds, often being combined with elderflower and peppermint in feverish states. It was also a valued remedy in high blood pressure and could be helpful in cystitis. Thus far everything was intelligible, but the words used to describe the herb's medicinal actions were a different matter. Yarrow was "diaphoretic, astringent, antipyretic, hypotensive and diuretic". I had to turn to the index at the end of the book to make sense of them, grasping as I did so that these were terms I would have to become fluent in.

I opened Dr Coffin's book, curious about what I was going to find. The book was a 40th edition, so it must have been in print, and popular, for many years. It was obvious that Dr Coffin had been held in high esteem, though, as I read on, I got the feeling that he can't have been an easy man to deal with. In classic Victorian manner, he held forth, dispensing knowledge of herbal medicine in a style that to the modern reader seemed overbearing and at times patronising. I thumbed through till I found the section on yarrow and read with interest.

Yarrow was diaphoretic, tonic, diuretic and a good wound healer, not too different from *Welsh Herbal Medicine*, it seemed. However, much of the section recounted the anecdote of an itinerant Quaker giving a talk about herbal medicine, presumably sometime in the early 19th century. When the speaker finished his talk, he was asked what he'd recommend to cure a common cold. "Take a pint of Yarrow tea made strong, on going to bed, and put a hot brick to thy feet …" he suggested.

The next question was on treatments for rheumatism. Without hesitation, the speaker responded with the exact same words: "Take a pint of Yarrow tea made strong, on going to bed, and …" And then, on being further questioned about expelling worms from children, his recommendation was: "Give them a strong Yarrow tea and put a warm brick to the feet, and they will be cured speedily."

Yarrow was evidently a 'cure all' for this speaker, though what the audience thought is not recorded. Dr Coffin had included the story in his book, so doubtless he considered yarrow to be a 'cure all' too. I didn't think this story would fit with my homework, but it was a window into a world where only the wealthy could afford a doctor, while herbal medicine was accessible to all.

* * *

Mike and I left early on Monday morning. Just after sunrise, I had carefully unearthed the roots of a yarrow growing by the front door and sealed the plant in a moist plastic bag. I hoped it would survive until I could press it. We were silent for much of the journey, but it was the silence of good friends—we'd had good talks, got plenty of 'miles in', and now we were on our way back to the demands of daily life. I dropped Mike outside his new studio, resisting the invite for a tour, and headed off to pick up Euan from nursery.

We went for a walk beside the canal and played games along the path. Vicki got back from college early and we had a relaxed supper together, chatting about our different weekends. I put Euan to bed, read him a story and then set about pressing the yarrow. It was fine and hadn't drooped. I pressed it between blotting paper and carefully placed it in the airing cupboard, weighing it down with books. I prayed it would be fully dry in two weeks, so that I could mount it and finish the Herbarium on time.

* * *

The School was in a substantial two-storey Arts and Crafts-style house to the south of the town, red brick and pebbledash, with painted wooden frames on large bay windows that rose to the full height of the building, each to one side of an arched entrance way with a heavy oak door. I rang the bell, knowing that I was early, perhaps too early, a shiver down my spine warning me that this was a consequential day in my life.

The door was opened by a young woman in a baggy jumper and jeans. She beckoned me to come in and welcomed me. A final-year student in charge of induction, she gave me sheaves of paper and course notes and told me where everything was. The School, including the classrooms, the secretary's office, kitchen and common room, was on the ground floor, she explained, and Mr van der Zee, the Principal, and his family lived on the first floor.

I found a desk in the classroom, sat down, and smiled at the few students who had already arrived. We were all looking at the paperwork with a mixture of excitement and dread. Reading lists and deadlines for submitting coursework for each module were laid out for the next twelve months: Introduction to Human Anatomy and Physiology, Biochemistry, Botany and Pharmacognosy, and Introduction to Herbal Medicine. At least there were no exams until the end of the second year.

The classroom filled up, and a ginger-haired man maybe ten years older than me sat down next to me and introduced himself. Dominic seemed to know a lot more about herbal medicine than me and had been planning to enrol on the course for the past two years. We talked away until Gus van der Zee walked into the room up to the blackboard and asked for silence.

He was a short, dapper man with greying hair and a neatly trimmed moustache, dressed in a dark, slightly creased suit. "Good morning, students," he started, his Flemish accent immediately apparent. Rocking up and down on his heels and toes, he welcomed us to the School, hoped we would find our studies rewarding and explained the week's timetable, running through the tutors taking each class.

Someone asked a question about the timetable, and it was clear he preferred not to be interrupted, though when he'd finished his introduction, he answered questions with good humour and a twinkle to his eyes. His eyes roved over this new bunch of students before him, assessing us as best he could. Twenty-five of us in the classroom, slightly more men than women, and the year's total intake just over one hundred. I didn't know it at the time but the attrition rate for the distance learning course was horrendous. Fifteen of us from the hundred managed to graduate at the end of four years—the course was a marathon, not a sprint.

The week went quickly, so much to learn and so little time. I began to realise that to practise herbal medicine well you needed an extraordinarily wide set of skills. I handed in my project and learnt that over the coming year I needed to do a further five native herbs to complete the Herbarium. I got to know fellow students in the kitchen or common room, or standing out in the garden—to my amazement quite a number still smoked. We swapped phone numbers and promised to stay in contact and support each other in the long months between the weeks at the School.

Mr van der Zee took two afternoon classes on herbal medicine. He was an entertaining teacher and it was a pleasure to sit there, listen and take notes. As a young man and a dairy farmer in Belgium, he'd routinely treated his cattle with herbal, rather than chemical, medicines and found them to be more effective and gentler than standard veterinary medicines. In the late 1960s, he'd sold up and moved to England to train as a medical herbalist. A lot of what he talked about came from his experience in herbal practice.

He explained that in popular herbal or folk medicine herbs were directly linked with specific disorders or illnesses: hops was a sleep aid for insomnia, elderflower was taken for catarrhal states of the nose and throat, such as colds and sinus problems. This unsophisticated approach, though clearly valuable, was quite distinct from the practice of scientifically based herbal medicine, known also as phytotherapy.

The scientific study of herbal medicines and their active ingredients led to an understanding of how a plant achieved its therapeutic effect. Often this approach confirmed the traditional use of a herb. Current research into rosemary showed that key active constituents improved memory and mental alertness. Traditional use of the herb as a warming tonic to aid memory went back for thousands of years—students in ancient Greece used rosemary when taking exams. It was no surprise to learn therefore that students taking the School's exams could also be found with flasks of rosemary tea on their desks.

He finished the class by handing out a two-page list of key words that we should memorise as soon as possible and suggested, with a droll look, that rosemary tea might help. I was right—here was the list of medicinal actions of plants that I had turned to in *Welsh Herbal Medicine*, except that this was twice the length—it started with 'antacid' and 'anti-allergy', through 'diaphoretic' and 'emmenagogue' and ended with 'thymoleptic' and 'vulnerary'.

Through learning these therapeutic actions, Mr van der Zee explained, it was possible to gain an awareness of the complexity inherent in plant medicines and, crucially, to differentiate between apparently similar herbs. For example, both calendula and yarrow were effective wound healers for cuts, abrasions and minor burns, but while calendula was antibacterial and anti-inflammatory, yarrow was astringent and anti-haemorrhagic. With this information you might choose to use calendula, where there was a risk of infection, and yarrow, where you wanted to protect and tighten tissue and staunch bleeding.

The class was over and Mr van der Zee wished us well in our studies. We had reached the end of an exciting but exhausting week, with new friends and newly acquired knowledge. I left for home with a clear view of what the course entailed and of the mountain I was aiming to climb.

Robin Nielsen

On the distance-learning course at the School, I would send off monthly written assignments on everything from Differential Diagnosis to Patho-physiology, Posology to Therapeutics. All went by post to the tutor concerned, and usually the work would come back, again by post, marked and with comments, within three weeks. Many tutors gave just a tick and a percentage mark at the end of the essay. A high mark might be gratifying, but it was feedback we wanted more than anything—a distance learning course involves hard, isolated work. Even mistakes (and ensuing criticism) affirmed a connection of sorts with the professional world of herbal medicine that we so avidly aspired to.

Robin Nielsen had small spidery handwriting and wrote in green ink. His comments tended to spread snakelike across the bottom of the page, or would burst out of the margins, and were often hard to decipher. Nevertheless, his comments on Therapeutics assignments were of a different order to those of most other tutors. You could tell that he had put thought and time into reading the important sections of the assignment and did his best to provide critical feedback and practical advice.

When I suggested in one assignment that thyme, liquorice and elecampane were the most useful herbs for chronic bronchitis, he explained that it was important to distinguish between 'wet' and 'dry' bronchitis.

In the former, where there was excess mucus production, astringent, drying herbs, such as ephedra and white horehound, were required that would control mucus production and stimulate the coughing up and clearance of phlegm.

Conversely, in 'dry' bronchitis, inflammation and a lack of lubricating mucus meant that a dry irritable cough was often present and that breathing could be strained and painful. This required herbs with a demulcent action, such as marshmallow and pleurisy root, that would moisten and soothe mucous membranes throughout the respiratory tract and lungs, and thus ease breathing.

I realised even then as a student that to the casual reader who knew nothing about herbal medicine such terms as 'wet' and 'dry' bronchitis taken on their own, might seem hopelessly naïve and unscientific. Yet they describe real-life scenarios and point to specific herbal medicines that will often prove effective. Too much knowledge, I thought to myself, may obscure simple solutions.

I knew that Robin was half Norwegian, but I never had the good fortune to meet him, as he retired shortly after I started practising in 1987. He was one of the stalwarts of British herbal medicine in the 20th century, when many thought that with the launch of the NHS in 1948, the profession of medical herbalism would slowly dwindle and disappear. At that time there were fewer than 100 herbal practitioners working in the entire country. Thankfully, that number was now creeping up again, and I and my fellow students represented a new wave of entrants to the profession, akin to the growth of the ecological and environmental movement, which saw herbal therapeutics as having a legitimate and valued place within the broad scope of medicine.

The Cat and Mutton

I was fortunate I didn't have to commute or stay in a dingy guest house. Having lived in Kent as a teenager, I had several friends I'd kept up with who were willing to put me up and lived close to Tunbridge Wells and the School of Herbal Medicine. The week-long study sessions were intensive and draining but that didn't stop me from being a bit of a lad again after the classes had finished in the evening. As teenagers, we'd hung out together, and zoomed around the countryside on our scooters, so, when we met up again, we'd relive old times, have a laugh and a beer and probably watch a movie or football. I saw The Blues Brothers for the first time at Phil's.

Phil was a kind man and, unlike most other friends, was curious about my studies and used to quiz me about what I'd learnt that day, sometimes asking me for my advice—did I know anything to treat verrucas or what could help with acid indigestion. He'd been brought up a Christian Scientist, so had an ambiguous attitude towards conventional medical care. He worked in the environmental health department at the local Council and his small, terraced house was always immaculate.

I didn't hear from him for a while and discovered from a mutual friend, Alan, that he'd fallen head over heels in love and was getting married in the spring. Phil had never seemed to have much luck with women, so I was happy for him. He had always wanted a lifelong partner. Alan had met Catrina, Phil's fiancée, and said they looked a good pair—she was a beautician, dark-haired, lively and attractive and Phil was a different person. Gone were those morose days when hardly a smile crossed his face.

Catrina moved in with Phil and I didn't like to impose on them. I stayed with other friends and saw Phil and Catrina occasionally but didn't keep up with them. As my studies deepened, I grew more and more involved in them and socialised less. After work each day, I studied for as many hours as I could, using holiday time for the week-long study sessions—what free time there was, was spent with family.

Quite out of the blue, Phil phoned me one evening, sounding stressed. Could he come and see me? He hoped I would be able to help him, but he didn't want to talk about it on the phone. I was free that Saturday, so invited him to come for supper and stay the night, and we could go down to the local pub and chat. He sounded relieved and said he looked forward to seeing us all. I had no idea what Phil wanted to talk about but imagined it was some kind of health problem. I hoped he hadn't been diagnosed with something serious.

Phil turned up on the dot and we had a pleasant meal, though I could see he was itching to talk to me. When we'd finished, I suggested we walk down through Broadway Market to the Cat and Mutton. Walking through the East End streets, Phil was shocked at the dilapidation and chaos—graffiti on the corrugated iron fencing of the building sites, and on the empty, vandalised shops. It was almost as if nothing had happened in the forty years since the Blitz.

One large wall had "Broadway Market is not a Sinking Ship, it's a Submarine" sprayed across it in capital letters—sometimes graffiti artists get it right! We walked into the Cat and Mutton, a down-at-heel, mostly friendly, Hackney pub and ordered our pints. No one took any notice of us, and we sat at a table by the window looking out in the dark across London Fields.

We sat quietly for a while and eventually I said, "Phil, you wanted to talk to me about something—I hope I can help."

Phil looked at me and his face creased in pain, "Catrina's walked out on me and she's not coming back. I gave her everything."

It all came pouring out. She hadn't been good with money and it had led to rows that had got increasingly heated, to the point where they had started throwing things at each other. One day he came back from work and she'd gone, with all her clothes and possessions, and their joint bank account emptied.

I felt deeply sorry for Phil and could see how wounded he was, but I couldn't quite understand why he had come to see me. I was more than happy to talk and help him as much as I could, but I knew he had good friends who lived close by, who would be willing to support and help him as needed.

"The thing is, Tom", he said, "I've decided I want to end it all, I can't cope with all this pain, I don't want to live any more—I thought you might be able to help, give me something to take. You know a poisonous herbal extract or root that I could eat or drink."

I looked at him in disbelief. No, this could not be, but it was—he was being completely serious. He had picked up enough knowledge from me of herbal medicine to understand that a medicine was a medicine at the correct dose but a poison in excess. One night after School, I'd talked to him about deadly nightshade and lily of the valley. That day in class we'd studied the strict prescribing and dosage regimes of toxic herbs that medical herbalists can use at low dosage, and Phil had paid close attention.

I didn't know what to say and took another sip from the glass. Phil was looking at me expectantly.

"Well, Phil", I said, "like everyone, when life has been too much there have been times when I've felt like ending it all, but I've always thought of those things that I really wanted to do and hadn't ever got round to doing. I don't know, things like going scuba diving in the Great Barrier Reef, or flying to Rio on Concorde, or going on a road trip across the US." I was struggling to come up with more examples, but I could see that I was getting somewhere and that Phil was engaged and thinking about what he hadn't done and might still like to do.

I watched and waited, wondering what he would come out with.

"Tom, you are quite right, there is something that I've never done and always meant to do."

I was all ears, what was he going to say?

"You know, I've never seen Crystal Palace play at home!"

I wasn't sure whether I was going to laugh or cry. I pulled myself together and said that this was just the one thing he could think of now, there would be lots of other things he could think of over time. In any case, the pain he was going through now wouldn't last forever—he had to look to the future and remember all the good things he had in his life, his work, his house, good friends, his parents.

We carried on chatting quietly and when we'd finished our drinks, Phil said, "Thanks Tom, I think you've helped me turn the corner. I'm going to go home tonight rather than stay with you. I have got to look to the future and get my life back again. Don't worry, I think I'm going to be alright."

We retraced our steps back through the ill-lit streets and gave each other a hug when we reached his car. He climbed in, gave me a determined look and, with a wave, set off towards the Blackwall Tunnel and the road back home.

Learning the craft

Two years into the course and I'd got into typical student habits again, skipping the odd piece of work or freewheeling—mostly due to lack of time or energy but occasionally when the motivation was lacking. There was such a vast amount to learn and so little time to process and absorb it, at times it felt impossible to take more in and integrate it effectively.

I passed the second-year exams without too much problem, thanks mostly to the revision classes that several of us had organised—meeting up on Sundays shortly before the exams—and reckoned that I knew the course material reasonably well, despite there being so many unanswered questions and, always, areas that could be explored in more depth.

My meeting with Dominic that first day at School was providential and had grown into a friendship. We regularly helped each other with assignments and, as I got to know him better, I discovered that he had been passionate about herbal medicine for years. A desk and two chairs sat in a small room in his house in St Albans, with dried herbs, tincture bottles and books on herbal medicine arranged along one of the walls. It didn't take me long to realise that he was quietly treating friends, family and neighbours with herbs, and that this had probably been going on for some while.

Dominic was divorced and had a five-year-old daughter, Frances, two years older than Euan, who lived with her mother most of the week. It turned out that Frances and Euan got on well, so on weekends when Frances was at Dominic's, we sometimes met up.

One weekend, while the children played in the garden, Dominic finally opened up and told me that three years ago he had sold his artists' materials supply business and was still living on the proceeds. What came next was a shock and unexpected—he'd sold the business because he had been diagnosed with non-Hodgkin's lymphoma.

Running the business had been stressful and overwhelming, to the point where his immune system must have crashed and opened the way for the cancer. He realised that if he wanted to recover, he had to sell the business and concentrate his energies on getting well again. He researched far and wide for information on herbal medicines, supplements and dietary regimes that might help, and decided to hold off taking chemotherapy until he could see whether natural treatments would work on their own.

He went on a strict exclusion diet, took lots of supplements and made-up prescriptions that included herbs such as barberry and poke root. Physician heal thyself, I mused, feeling humbled. He wasn't sure it was going to work to begin with but he got the all-clear after eight months and now had regular six-monthly check-ups. He was sure it wouldn't be coming back. No wonder he had the confidence to give herbal medicine to would-be patients, I thought—contrary, of course, to School regulations.

With Dominic's help I acquired the basics to produce my own tinctures and make simple creams and ointments. I bought several large glass jars from him and, using 40% vodka, made tinctures of fresh plantain, rosemary and sage from my garden, pressing them after ten days with a wine press, bottling and labelling them and placing them alongside the dried herbs and tinctures already on the shelf—the beginnings of my own dispensary!

Clinical training commenced at the start of the third year, and the emphasis of the course changed entirely. We were trainees now, apprentices learning the craft, working with real patients with real illnesses. It dawned on us that staff at the School and tutors in the clinic treated us differently—we were prospective practitioners now, rather than students.

The clinic was in a quiet neighbourhood in Balham, south London, not too far from the Underground station. Dressed in our stiff new white coats, we sat in upright chairs round the edge of the consulting room that doubled as a classroom when no patients were present, with a mix of discomfort and anticipation.

It was 9am on a Saturday morning, a busy day at the clinic, and the tutor—Brian Davies, an experienced practitioner and former biology teacher—cantered through the clinic rules and routines, with our first patient due at 9.30am for an hour-long appointment:

"The needs and sensibilities of patients come first," he said with emphasis, "despite the fact that this is a teaching clinic. No student is allowed to give advice to a patient without the express consent of a tutor—this applies throughout the building, in reception, in the waiting room, in the clinic room and in the dispensary.

"You must arrive on time … In certain situations, the tutor may need to see the patient on their own. There will be no talking during a consultation and nothing done to distract the patient, tutor or student taking the case history …"

It seemed a lot at the time, though it was all common sense. There was more to come—including the rota for cleaning the kitchen and bathroom—but he would explain this during the lunch break.

Our first patient was an elderly woman with rheumatoid arthritis, accompanied by her daughter. Bent over and walking with a stick, the lady moved painfully across the room, sitting down cautiously in the chair. She was 78 and had had rheumatoid arthritis for nearly a year. The anti-inflammatories she was taking were helping but perhaps herbal medicine might ease the pain a little more and help her to live more independently?

Brian sat there, giving his full attention to mother and daughter, putting them at ease, despite the six students in white coats hanging on every word on the far side of the room! He carefully included the daughter in the conversation, encouraging her to join in. We could all see that her mother was trying to make light of her symptoms. Yes, she admitted, it was affecting her sleep, she was woken several times a night by the pain, which was worst in her hands and feet. It was difficult to find a comfortable position.

Brian teased out more and more information, and it became clear that the most pressing problem was in her hands—she found it difficult to cut up food or lift heavy pans or plates. At the end of the session, after examining her joints and taking her pulse and blood pressure, he turned towards us and asked if anyone had any questions.

Ceri, who was an auxiliary nurse and always seemed one step ahead of the rest of us, asked astutely, could she dress herself in the morning and make her own breakfast? This gained an appreciative nod from the daughter. It could take half an hour to get dressed in the morning, was the reluctant reply, and sometimes she had just toast for breakfast.

When they had left the room, Brian gave a summary of the case and his initial thoughts on treatment, quizzed us briefly on the key signs and symptoms of RA and its differential diagnosis, and discussed herbs that he thought should be included in the prescription. Which herb was most strongly indicated and what about topical treatment, he asked. We all knew devil's claw root was specific for RA but what were its potential side effects?

As usual Dominic was first to answer—as a strong bitter devil's claw could cause stomach irritation, so it was best to prescribe it along with other anti-inflammatories, such as meadowsweet and liquorice, which protected the stomach mucosa. As for local treatment, how about comfrey leaf oil with essential oils of lavender and wintergreen? Dominic was just a bit too eager, I thought, but his suggestions couldn't be faulted. After more discussion, Brian finalised the prescription and took it off to be dispensed.

We saw eight patients during that first day, and when there were gaps, discussed cases that we'd seen and practised taking blood pressure. It was a long day, and sitting on the Tube on the journey back home, I reflected that clinical training was a mighty challenge. There were no limits to the skills required to treat patients successfully or to match patients with effective treatment.

We role-played, playing 'practitioner' and 'patient' with each other and then reversing roles. To start with it seemed so difficult to find the right words as the 'practitioner', even Ceri, had awkward pauses. Playing the 'patient' was easier, but this was deceptive: you soon became aware of just how focused and attuned a practitioner needed to be—one misstep and you could undermine the patient's confidence in you (and your confidence in yourself).

The case history form that listed key areas for questioning and note taking, such as childhood illnesses, familial health problems and current medication, helped to keep us on track. If you lost your way and ground to a halt, you could pretend to study the notes, glossing over the awkwardness and buying yourself time to come up with a new line of questioning.

Eventually, everyone had to push through their fears and take a patient for a standard thirty-minute appointment. Brian, or Margaret Butterworth, who took over when Brian was away, sat close by, observing and ready to support or intervene as needed.

I got off lightly with my first patient—a 15-year-old boy with acne, who came with his mother. The boy's symptoms had been steadily improving over the months he had been attending the clinic. Both were positive about the treatment and did their best to help me keep focused and steer my way through the consultation—all I had to do was examine his skin, ask obvious questions and say that, subject to Brian's agreement, he should continue with the existing treatment.

Other students were not so fortunate, finding that patients who were desperate or indifferent to the plight of the student, could just ignore them—leaving them stranded—and direct all their attention towards the tutor.

Our progress at the clinic was matched by a different focus at School. Now we studied Differential Diagnosis, Clinical Skills, Pharmacology, Pharmacy and Herbal Therapeutics—subjects essential to safe and effective practice. While we practised specific clinical routines at the clinic, such as the cardio-vascular system, at the School we were able to connect these routines more directly with the medical science that underpinned them.

Mr van der Zee was his usual entertaining self, teaching Herbal Therapeutics in the afternoon sessions. After a general introduction to the subject, he moved on to talk about dosage—a subject that had us all confused. Different authorities recommended widely different dosages for the same herbs. Mr van der Zee's answer to this was to give us a booklet listing the School's recommended dosages for well over a hundred medicinal plants. It included an additional section for those potentially poisonous herbs prescribed within precise, legally defined, doses.

The challenge, he said, when prescribing was to produce an effective combination of four or five herbs that was tailored to the specific state of the patient. By combining and blending different herbs together, a greater therapeutic effect could be achieved than resulted from using the same herbs individually on their own.

Although in practice this meant that herbs were rarely prescribed close to their maximum dosage, it was essential to know the minimum and maximum dosages of all the herbs on the list—we would be examined on them in both the written and clinical exams. The vast majority of medicinal herbs, he continued—with a look reminding us that certain herbs were lethal in excess—were sufficiently gentle in their action that even if the maximum dose was exceeded it was unlikely to lead to side effects.

Nevertheless, it was not enough to simply produce an accurate prescription. Clear instructions to the patient and clear thinking were of equal importance. As a practitioner, you could make up a perfect prescription and provide essential advice but if the patient did not comply, it might all be wasted effort.

With a laugh, he turned to talking about a patient who'd come to see him with digestive problems. She'd tried countless treatments and seen no benefit. He could see that she was determined to get well and instructed her to fast one day a fortnight, taking just two cloves of garlic during the day and drinking lots of water. For the rest of the time, he gave her a diet sheet and a prescription containing standard herbs for the condition: chamomile, cramp bark, valerian and peppermint.

She came back four weeks later much improved. Her digestion was far more comfortable and her bowels were controlled and more or less regular. The only problem, she said, was that her husband had complained vociferously about the strong smell of garlic that emanated from her for several days after each fast.

Pleased with the outcome, Mr van der Zee presumed that her husband had simply been over-sensitive about the garlic. At this point, he seemed barely able to prevent himself from laughing out loud, as he had then discovered that she had been taking two *heads* of garlic a day—perhaps twenty cloves—rather than the recommended two. He had felt rather foolish, but his patient was simply happy to be feeling so much better.

Here was an example of failing to give clear instructions to the patient, he said. Fortunately, in this case the outcome had been entirely positive and it led him to consider prescribing higher doses of garlic to patients, when indicated.

* * *

As we moved into the fourth and final year, I knew that however hard I tried, there was never going to be enough time each week to learn the year's material, let alone consolidate and integrate it all, in preparation for the exams. What with working full-time, looking after Euan, completing the monthly assignments and going to the clinic, spare time was almost non-existent.

Ultimately, this had led to the break-up of our relationship. Vicki lived a busy life too, teaching at college and campaigning on environmental and women's issues. Over the years, we set aside less and less time to be together, each over-committed, until—and despite the joy Euan brought us—we grew far apart and eventually separated. I moved out and rented a room in a friend's flat a short walk away and continued looking after Euan two to three days a week, though now he had to share my room and sleep on a sofa-bed.

I tried to see if I could reduce my hours at the housing association but there was little flexibility. A group of twelve of us organised Sunday sessions once a month, bringing in experienced tutors—medical and herbal practitioners—to teach their specialist clinical areas, such as gynaecology and paediatrics, and to hone our practical skills in advance of the final clinical exam in December.

By June I knew I was falling behind and couldn't see how I could complete the course and at the same time revise sufficiently. I was aware too that failing the written exams in September barred you from sitting the clinical exam in December. Normally cautious, I took the plunge and handed in my notice at the housing association.

I revised solidly for eight weeks and finally felt on top of it all. I wrote notes on index cards using coloured inks to highlight different features of exam questions and the clinical exam routines, and went through them every night before going to bed. By the time the written exams came round, I felt confident.

The exams were held in the School, and we all feared our car would break down or something would stop us arriving on time. Dominic and I decided to drive in convoy, so if the worst happened, we could abandon one of the cars. Driving down the A21 at 8am the morning of the first exam my car stalled and wouldn't start again—I drifted onto the hard shoulder, trying and trying to start the engine again. Dominic reversed back till he was parked in front of my little Fiat, came over and peeked through the window.

"Give it one more go," he said. Miraculously the engine took this time, and we were off again.

The exams were almost a relief—I had prepared well and wrote at length, having predicted fairly clearly what questions would come up.

It was a long six weeks till the results were out but Dominic and I had both managed to achieve good grades.

* * *

I arrived at the clinic in Balham in good time. Waiting in the reception area, where our patients routinely sat, I was abuzz, my heart racing—so much hung on passing this exam. It was early December and, under my breath, I found myself humming the tune to the carol *See Amid the Winter Snow*. It came to me that I hadn't been this nervous since I was 12 and had sung this as a duet in the school carol service.

In the event, all went well. My patient had had shingles on her scalp and forehead. She was past the infectious stage and the blistering had not spread down to her eye, though she was left with chronic pain where the infection had taken root—post-herpetic neuralgia. The consultation went smoothly, I felt confident and managed to cover all the essential questioning and to relate to the patient in a relaxed manner.

After twenty minutes the examiners—two senior herbalists and a practising GP—interrupted me and asked me to examine the peripheral nervous system on the patient, testing the sensory and motor function of her arms and legs. Once she had left the room, they quizzed me on the cranial nerves, their distribution and common pathologies associated with them.

Next, I was given five minutes to draw up a treatment plan for her—a herbal prescription, dietary advice and other recommendations. Why had I chosen these specific herbs, what side effects or interactions were associated with them? Was I confident that I had prescribed the herbs at an appropriate dosage? How much, if any, improvement would I expect to see in the patient's symptoms in two weeks' time?

That the examiners were relaxed and smiling as I left the room was a good sign, but there were three nervous weeks to wait for the official results. If I had passed, I would begin practising in the new year.

First do no harm

Like many new-qualified practitioners, I started out by being over-familiar with my patients. I didn't realise that being caring and attentive was not the same as treating patients as friends.

About six months into practice, a young woman in her late twenties came to see me with chronic pains in her abdomen—a difficult condition to make sense of and diagnose. I quizzed her closely, and as we talked, I began to suspect that she had irritable bowel syndrome and that her symptoms were linked to her menstrual cycle and a pattern of mood swings that veered from elation to near despair. I took her pulse, looked at her tongue and palpated her abdomen—all were normal. Eventually, I prescribed her angelica root, cramp bark and white peony, herbs that would be warming and relaxant, and support hormonal and emotional balance.

Over several months, her symptoms lessened but did not altogether go away, though overall she felt healthier and more stable. We developed a friendly, bantering relationship during the half-hour appointments. Sometimes we spoke to each other in a rather tongue-in-cheek way, each saying mildly silly or outrageous things, knowing that they were not meant and that there was a kind of intimacy in this fooling around.

After a long wait, she was given a date for hospital investigations to try to get to the root of the abdominal pains. She would be an in-patient for two days and had been told that she couldn't take her herbal medication with her. This was standard hospital procedure but in the way she said it, there was an undercurrent of complaint, perhaps of challenge. Wanting to be helpful and responding subliminally to that hint of challenge, I offered to visit her in hospital and bring her herbal prescription with me. She thought that was a great idea. and I arranged to see her on the ward on the Saturday, her second day in hospital.

After following the signs along a maze of corridors, I pushed my way through the swing doors and found her sitting up in bed reading. She was in a small ward with two other female patients. She looked tired.

"It's a challenge sleeping in here," she said, as she closed the book.

"You do look a bit pale."

"Oh, I'm fading away, almost at death's door. I've had lots of blood taken from both arms," she said, opening out her arms and showing me purple black bruises on the inside of each elbow.

"Of course, you've had pints of blood taken," I replied, "you poor thing. And now you're going to tell me that they're quietly starving you."

"How did you know that? Do you know what lunch was today …?"

We carried on in this light-hearted vein, batting jokey comments back and forth, until I remembered that I had her tincture in my rucksack. Pulling the dark glass bottle from the depths of the bag, I passed it over to her and said, "Here's your poison!"

It was a just a play on the word "potion" but, as the words left my mouth, I knew that I had crossed a line and said something unforgiveable. For the briefest second, a mixture of fear and horror flashed across her face, but she recovered quickly and, in a steady voice, said, "Thanks for bringing it in. Can you put it in a glass for me?"

I measured out a 5ml teaspoonful of tincture, added water and gave it to her. She sipped it slowly.

"It doesn't taste any better than the last bottle," she said, breaking the silence. I was still shocked by what I'd said and didn't reply.

"Really, I should be happy," she continued. "They haven't found anything wrong with me, despite all the blood tests and investigations. The other women here both have bowel cancer. It puts things in perspective, though I'd still like to know why I keep on getting the pains."

We talked for a while and she said she'd make an appointment to see me again after she'd seen the consultant. We said goodbyes and I found my way out of the hospital into the afternoon sunlight. It might have been 4 o'clock on the Euston Road, with traffic jams and fumes, but I took a deep breath in and inwardly berated myself and my uncontrolled tongue. How could I use such a word to describe a medicine? For several days, I relived the moment, as it played over in my mind.

She came to see me several weeks later with an inconclusive diagnosis of irritable bowel syndrome from the consultant. She laughed at how, after all that effort, she was back where she'd started. But her heart wasn't in it, and the lightness that had been a feature of our exchanges was gone. I suggested we try some new herbs and she agreed. At the end of the session she left with a wistful look, medicine in hand. She never returned.

* * *

This happened years ago, before I began fully to appreciate the power of the therapeutic relationship, both its strength and fragility. As I found out the hard way, a single misplaced word can simply dissolve what holds it together. Conversely, of course, a well-placed word may strengthen and transform it. Build it with care and attention, with a firm intent to 'first do no harm', and the therapeutic relationship can become a place of refuge and healing, where—like an opening door—hope and confidence can enter in.

Two years on

I was sitting on more or less the same chair at the front of the Conference room waiting for the AGM to begin. Out of the window, the clouds hung heavily over the garden with rhododendrons and azaleas in flower and the sea stretching beyond. The hotel, up on the cliffs overlooking Torbay, had been such a success for the 1987 Conference that everyone had voted to return again in two years' time.

Twenty minutes early and the room was still almost empty. I thought back to the moment two years ago, when the fifteen of us who had come through the exams had stood to take the Hippocratic oath and then filed up to the dais, where Council members sat, to receive our membership certificates from the President, each neatly rolled into a tube and tied with scarlet ribbon.

There was my name, when I opened it—Thomas Bretland—in black ink on cream card, beneath the Coat of Arms of the National Institute of Medical Herbalists. I sat back down and held on to it, as if it were a talisman.

This time round was different. Now I was in practice with a growing patient list, even if I was still struggling financially. Years ago I'd read that Arthur Conan-Doyle only turned to writing because he couldn't earn a living as a doctor. In a strange way, I took heart from this.

If doctors struggled to build a successful practice before the NHS existed, then taking a while to build a herbal practice was much to be expected.

I practised two days a week at the Islington Natural Health Centre in Highbury and was teaching an evening class in Herbal Medicine in central London. In January, I had been offered a job as a medical herbalist at Haggerston Health Group and now worked there one day a week. It was an exciting place to work, part funded by the NHS, it was a community project that provided a range of therapies at minimal cost, to people aged 55 and over living in Hackney.

The users, as the patients were known, mostly lived in high-rise blocks in council estates scattered across the borough. When I'd started, I'd wondered how they would respond to bitter-tasting tinctures and teas. True, there were a few who didn't come back after they'd tried their first prescription, but in general I could not have asked for more enthusiastic or committed patients.

Almost all of them were taking medication for high blood pressure and diabetes along with benzodiazepine tranquillisers, such as valium, to help with anxiety. I had to learn quickly about potential interactions and had a waiting list of patients who wanted to see me to help wean them off the tranquillisers. I'd thought that older patients might be more fussy but the reverse was the case—even small gains were appreciated.

Looking around, I saw Dominic and Lucy come in at the far end of room, and they gave me a wave. They'd become a fixture in the last year, at about the same time that Josie and I had moved in together. It was good to see them looking relaxed and happy—maybe Lucy would move in with Dominic and they would both practise together.

I watched as the room slowly filled up, an atmosphere building of quiet anticipation. Ceri came over and began telling me about an Ayurveda seminar she'd been to. She was full of it and it sounded very interesting. The tutor had been apprenticed as an Ayurvedic doctor at the age of six, which meant that he'd been in practice for over sixty years, she said, conveying genuine astonishment. He'd talked about 'embodied beings' and the 'doshas', and a range of Ayurvedic herbs, and it had all made so much sense. Once she'd finished telling me the story, she moved on to share it with Chris, who was sitting behind me.

On the raised tables in front of me, Council members were beginning to take their place. Julia Douglas-Smythe sat down more or less opposite me, and shortly after Bill Kersley sat down beside her. They started talking away, and I couldn't help hearing their conversation. Julia was about 75 and practised in a large house in Putney, near the river. It was said that her practice included aristocrats and royalty but I did know, from a friend who'd worked as her dispenser, that she had a very busy practice and that patients often left with carrier bags full of herbs and supplements.

While Julia was unconventional and eccentric, Bill, in his sixties, was perhaps the opposite. A Yorkshireman, with a long-established, successful practice in Bradford, he was a Baptist, fiercely proud of the Institute and committed to the professional development, and image, of medical herbalism. He was probably the only herbalist in the country who drove a brand-new Jaguar. He wanted to show the world that herbalists could be successful and that they had to be reckoned with.

They talked away, and I listened to their conversation with increasing amazement. They were quietly competing with each other.

"So, how many patients died in your consulting room this year?" asked Julia, as if this was an everyday event.

"Oh, this year I had three patients die in the waiting room, and with one of them I had to wait until the police doctor arrived and examined him," replied Bill, almost nonchalantly. Julia looked a bit put out but she wasn't going to let Bill get away with this.

"Well, I had one in the waiting room and one on the couch," said Julia, with the slightest hint of satisfaction.

Bill was on the point of continuing the conversation when the President stood up, cleared his throat, and called the meeting to order, leaving me aghast, and unable to believe what I had just heard. This was another world, far beyond my experience. I had so much to learn— Life is short, the Art is long, I whispered to myself.

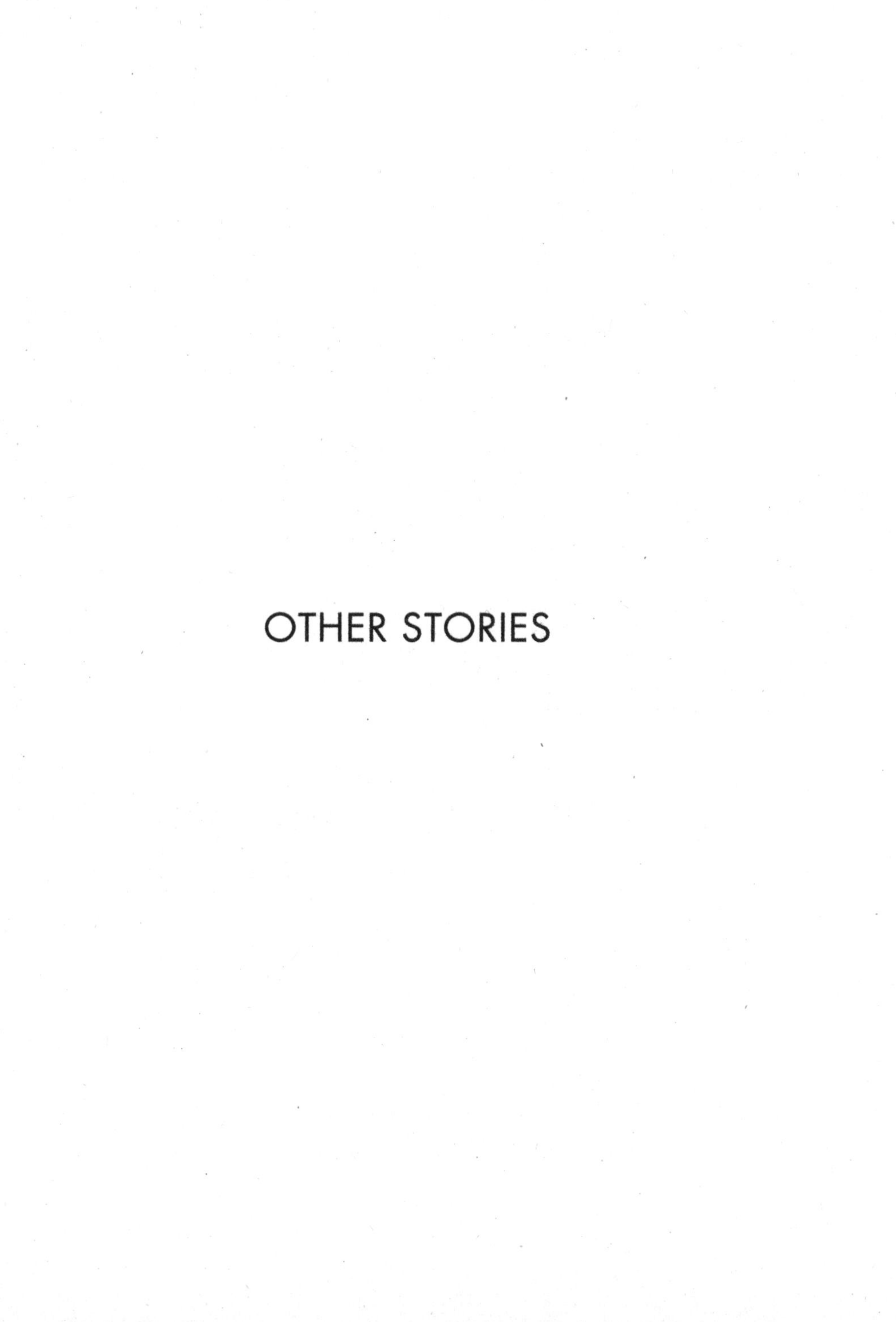

OTHER STORIES

Nathan

Nathan came to see me about seven years ago suffering with anxiety and recurrent migraines. Quick-witted and perceptive but with a sharp tongue and a sarcastic turn of phrase, he was leaning back casually, one arm draped over the back of the chair, looking me straight in the eyes. In his early twenties, I got the sense he could make enemies as easily as friends.

"So, herbal medicine works, yeah? What do you think you can do for me?"

"That all depends on you," I said, somehow finding the right words in response. "I can give you herbs that will help you to relax and to control your symptoms, but they will work significantly better if you also follow the advice I'm going to give you."

He paused, and I could see him going over what I'd just said. A half-smile flitted across his face and he said, "OK, ask away, let me know what I'm in for!"

First test passed, I thought. The next test would be making recommendations that were realistic for his student lifestyle. He was a fashion student at the University of the Arts, London but you wouldn't have known it—he was sitting there unshaved, in a red check shirt, jeans and sandals with socks. His stamina and energy levels were good, he went swimming twice a week. Food, study, alcohol and sleep all happened at some point each day, though in variable quantities and often, it seemed, not in that order.

On a hunch, I asked if he was a perfectionist, and he gave me a caustic look, as if to say, so you've finally worked that out, and replied with a laugh, "Don't you know I'm a tortured soul who hates to fail?"

I gave him a diet sheet with "Eat food, not too much, mostly vegetables" underlined at the top. "You want to eat food close to its natural state," I explained. "You need to avoid foods with added sugar and ultra-processed foods—these are pro-inflammatory and will contribute to triggering headaches and migraine. You could try cutting out dairy produce for a couple of weeks and see if this makes a difference. You *must* drink more water, just being dehydrated can bring on anxiety and headaches."

That was enough, I said to myself—overload him with advice and he'll give up and walk away. I prescribed him valerian tablets and a tincture containing chamomile, feverfew and skullcap, and he left looking positive and engaged.

He came back three weeks later looking more relaxed and without the angry undertone that had been there before. He had managed to take the herbs well, eaten more carefully and drunk plenty of water. He'd had just one migraine, which had been mild, and overall he felt better, though whether this was down to the herbs or not, he couldn't say. I agreed—ascribing benefit to a treatment is difficult—and suggested that he carry on with his new routine and take the herbs for a further three or four weeks.

I didn't see him again until the following spring, when he came to see me a month or so before his finals. He was getting nervous about the exams, he said, and this was affecting his memory and sleep. He was awake at 4am each morning and couldn't get back to sleep. Eventually, he admitted that the real problem was that he had just split up with his girlfriend of four years, and that this is what was stressing him. He was well ahead in completing the designs for his clothes and, as long as he was sleeping well, he should be fine revising and with the exams.

I suggested he do deep breathing exercises, when he got into bed and if he woke during the night and couldn't get back to sleep. This could be very relaxing and aid sleep. He should start taking the valerian tablets again, alongside ashwagandha powder at one level teaspoonful twice a day. This should be enough to restore his sleep pattern and would have a calming effect.

Several months on, I discovered that Nathan had got a First in his exams and his designs had caused quite a stir on the catwalk. They had been described as 'simultaneously provocative and discreet', and he'd gone on to win *The Guardian's* 'Young Fashion Designer of the Year' award. His clothes had got a lot of social media coverage and he'd been headhunted by a fashion house in New York—he was leaving for the US later that month. I felt glad for him and didn't expect to hear from him again.

Sitting in the kitchen a few weeks later at around 10pm, I got a call from a US number. It was Nathan phoning from New York. Could he talk to me? He was very apologetic for calling so late but he couldn't call while he was at work. I did my best to put on a reassuring voice and let him talk away.

At first, when he won the award, it had been very exciting. He'd been widely congratulated for his original work and there was lots of media interest. Several well-known fashion brands had contacted him with offers of in-house work. Carried away by the attention and celebrity status that went with the prize, he'd accepted this high-powered job in New York, though it meant long hours and lots of pressure.

It wasn't working out as he'd hoped—he felt boxed in and perhaps he wasn't ready to make the kind of commitment expected of him. He had thought long and hard about what to do and who to contact for advice—what did I think he should do?

Great Nathan, thanks for putting me on the spot, I said quietly to myself. There was no answer to his question. I couldn't tell him what he should do, and there was no way of knowing what was the right choice for him.

Easy decisions are ones where it's 65% in favour vs 35% against. When the odds are as clear as this, the decision stares you in the face. But where the odds are 52% vs 48%, decision-making can become agony, as—stuck in the jaws of ambivalence—you swing from one decision to the other. The only way out of this painful place is, I believe, to reflect long and hard and then—one way or another—make a *wholehearted* decision. When you have done everything possible to make the right decision, at least—and this is very important—you cannot blame yourself should things go wrong. Unfortunately, I didn't think this was what Nathan wanted to hear.

A distant memory insinuated itself in my mind—how it arrived, I have no idea, but it could not have been more apt. A winter's day in the college library reading in the warmth, while the rain poured out-side. I was looking at a short pamphlet by Jean-Paul Sartre and had been struck by its acute intelligence. During the German occupation of France in 1940, a student of his had come to see him for advice. He wanted to join the Resistance and fight to liberate his country from tyranny but his mother was widowed and he was her only support. What should he do? Should he join the Resistance and abandon his mother, or look after his mother and give up on fighting the Nazis?

Sartre's reply surprised me and showed great subtlety: I cannot tell you what you should do, he said, but I can tell you that in coming to see me you had probably already formed an idea of what I would advise you to do. This is likely to be the best decision for you. The student realised there and then what he needed to do—to stay and support his mother. He thanked Sartre and left.

I followed Sartre's example and repeated his words to Nathan … I can't tell you what you should do, I said, but I can tell you that in phoning me you had probably already formed an idea of what I would advise you to do. This is likely to be the best decision for you.

Nathan was silent for a moment, and immediately began thanking me. He had realised in a flash what he should do, began saying his goodbyes, and without even telling me what decision he'd come to, put down the phone!

Just under a year later he came to see me, and I finally learnt that he had come back to London soon after our phone call. He was work-ing freelance and was a lot more self-assured, though still spiky. Over several years, he carried on coming to see me when needed for treat-ment or advice, not always being the best of patients and often being argumentative, until one day just as he was leaving, I could hold myself back no longer and told him that he needed *to be kind to himself.*

Perhaps, I shouldn't have said it, for he didn't respond, gave me a scathing look and headed out the door. That was the last time I saw him.

Chantin

"Hi Tom, I haven't seen you for ages, how are you?"

She was sitting on a bench on the seafront at Sheringham and I hadn't spotted her, had almost walked past. She was eating an ice cream and looking relaxed in tee shirt and jeans, long black hair done up loosely in a bun.

"Hi Chantin, how are you doing, nice ice cream? You're looking well." I meant it, she always seemed to radiate a sense of lightness and wellbeing.

"I'm fine, thanks—but you're looking a bit frazzled," she said, looking at me closely. She was right. I was stressed. I told her about the building works at home, and how the two days a week commute to work in London was becoming too much.

She smiled and rolled her eyes.

"When I first came to Europe everyone kept talking about 'stress' and I really hadn't a clue what they meant. I'd ask, 'What is this stress you're talking about?'"

She shrugged her shoulders to add emphasis, gesturing with palms up, eyes wide.

"And they'd look at me in disbelief—'How could you not know what stress is?'—but I really didn't, it was not something I'd ever experienced."

Chance meetings sometimes open up new worlds. I was drawn in and wanted to know more.

"I grew up in Kathmandu with brothers and sisters, aunts, uncles and cousins everywhere—even as a child I could walk around most of the city and know that relatives were close by. There was a sense too that everyone looked out for one another. People cared about each other, and though they could be sad or suffering, this was not a permanent state. Also, there was never a sense of time pressure, things happened at a human pace.

"When I came to university in London, life was completely different and many of my fellow students complained of stress and burn-out. I don't know, I've always danced, been a dancer, perhaps that's why I still didn't experience it.

"After graduation I started to tour all over Europe, often for weeks at a time. I am very fortunate because performing traditional Nepalese dance is basically a joy for me. You're expressing yourself all the time through your body (she was moving playfully and twisting her torso, as she spoke), expressing all the emotions from sadness to laughter—and being appreciated for it.

"Then one day, after many years, I was heading to Barcelona for a performance and had a plane to catch. We were on the motorway, well on schedule, all was fine. Then the traffic started queueing up ahead and we came to a standstill. I was still confident we'd make it, telling myself 'there's still plenty of time yet, no worries', but the traffic just stayed where it was. The minutes ticked by and the chances of making the flight got smaller and smaller.

"Then suddenly, sitting there in the car, I finally felt it—stress! Just as everyone had said: my heart was racing, I was hot and bothered and anxious, feeling trapped and sort of out of control—all those things I'd been told about over the years. I missed the flight and joined the world of stress!"

"I can't believe you lived in Europe so long without getting stressed," I said. "What about now—do you get stressed now?"

"Oh," she smiled ruefully, "I get stressed like everyone else. I suppose my mind and body learned the pattern that day on the motorway and now it just switches on when the pressure gets too much."

She glanced down at her watch, then back up at me with an apologetic look. "Nice to meet up with you, Tom, I've got to go now. Hope to see you again soon."

And she was off, back into the town.

Reading Signs

My aunt Sophie developed polymyalgia rheumatica in her late seventies and was prescribed high-dose steroids to control the inflammation. This did not stop her from travelling far and wide. She had been a diplomat and lived at different times in Bonn, Rangoon and Washington. Travel was in her blood and once retired she maintained a dizzying schedule of international flights and cruises, along with week-long art classes in Northumbria, the south of France and Morocco.

One day on a train back to London from Newcastle, being a naturally talkative person, she fell into conversation with the man opposite her across the table, a cardiac surgeon as it turned out. They talked away for a good while, about the state of the railways and the NHS, her art course in Northumberland and her painting, till there was a pause in the conversation, when with a certain edge of embarrassment, he asked, "I hope you don't mind me asking but you are taking steroids, aren't you?"

His surgeon's eye had noted the significant 'jowls' and broadened, flabby chin and neck that had changed her face over the previous few months, giving it a slightly bloated, puffy, appearance. From long experience, he had recognised this pattern as the result of long-term high-dose steroid intake and had wanted to confirm that his assessment was accurate.

Sophie was impressed and, several days later, enthusiastically recounted the story to me. It has stayed in my mind as an example of how careful observation and repeated exposure to particular signs can make identifying them more or less straightforward, though it can take years to become fluent in reading them.

For the herbalist, when starting out in practice, it can seem impossible to realise such a skill. People tend to consult medical herbalists with conditions like anxiety and poor sleep, eczema, migraine, irritable bowel syndrome, and chronic fatigue—(dys)functional conditions that lack clear diagnostic signs but are not life-threatening. Relatively few patients come with undiagnosed pathological conditions, such as Parkinson's disease or rheumatoid arthritis, conditions which over time reveal specific diagnostic signs.

If you aim as a practitioner to prevent illness and to maintain health, this means trying to work with subtle, hard-to-read signs that may only partially indicate underlying ill health, as many diagnostic signs only become apparent once serious illness has set in.

To work well as a medical herbalist then, it pays to become adept at 'fuzzy logic', at reading and interpreting subtle *patterns* of 'unwellness' along with specific clinical signs. These 'patterns' can be subliminal and are not always directly visible or accessible to the analytical mind: sometimes all that is present are facial and bodily expressions, a series of hints and nudges that taken together may indicate imbalance, emotional disturbance, organ weakness or a tendency towards specific types of ill health. Both analytical and intuitive minds need to be engaged.

Wonderfully vague, you may say! Yes, but this is what you have to deal with if you are aiming to prevent ill health *before* it manifests, before it becomes real and recognisable.

Developing the skill to read and interpret patterns of illness in a patient is like learning a new language. In point of fact, it is learning a new language. At first you work hard simply to decipher the most basic words and phrases, to recognise the most simple or common of signs, a slight tremor in the hand or facial flushing, for example. You have to learn a whole new vocabulary. Though it is not a language that you can ever become entirely fluent in, those phrases and sentences that you do manage to catch give you a head start.

* * *

Having set myself on the path of learning to read this language as best I could, my fluency was one day put to the test, when I came down to reception to meet my next patient, Jim, who had recently arrived from Australia.

Working in a clinic with upstairs rooms can be a serious problem but it has one advantage—observing a patient navigate their way up and down stairs can tell you more about their health in seconds than fifteen minutes of talking.

Jim was sitting reading a magazine. Aged about 55, I thought, slightly flushed, balding and somewhat overweight, especially around the waist. We greeted each other—he was alert and intelligent with a cheerful, positive face, and we shook hands, his grip warm and friendly. It was a far cry from the unpleasant 'empty' hand of someone who wants to give nothing, and the vice-like grip of the hand that seeks to ensure that you know who is in control. He paused momentarily to recover his breath at the top of the stairs, and we went into the room and sat down.

He had just arrived in England—it was all new to him—and was starting a job in finance in Norwich the following Monday. His naturopath in Melbourne had recommended that he come and see me for ongoing treatment. The normal pleasantries and basic details completed—he was 53 years old and was renting a house near the university—he asked me how I worked. Did he need to get a range of blood tests before I could begin to treat him, as was the case with his naturopath?

I didn't know what to answer—this was not a question that had been put to me so directly before. Over the years I had become less reliant on getting blood tests from patients. If they had blood test results this was unquestionably useful, but my priority had been to develop the ability to assess a patient's state of health using careful observation—clinical signs, 'fuzzy' patterns and intuition—along with close, attentive listening and simple clinical examination skills, rather than to focus on standardised tests.

It was rare for me to ask patients to get blood tests, I explained, as I would suggest a visit to the GP, if I thought routine investigations, including blood tests, were needed. But how did I know what was wrong with someone or when to refer to a GP, he asked, without blood tests? He wasn't being difficult, this was how his naturopath worked and he couldn't see how I could work without them. I realised then that this was a test that had been waiting for me for a long time.

"I suppose the best way to describe how I work is like an old-fashioned GP," I said, "with accurate questioning, careful observation and some simple clinical examinations."

"OK," he said, "judging on what you can see and observe so far, what's wrong with me?"—meaning, you are observing me, what assessment have you made?

"Give me a few moments to work this out," I said, holding back the sense of panic and speeding heart rate developing in my chest. Could I really do this? Taking a deep breath and settling into my chair, I looked closely at him and drew together what I had observed so far, with what I could see now.

He carried significant weight around his abdomen—an indicator, I reminded myself, of overeating or poor diet, lack of exercise, chronic inflammation, impaired sugar control and raised cholesterol levels—and this was very obvious in comparison to other areas of his body, which were trim. His facial skin was greasy and slightly wrinkled, and there were early signs of an enlarging, reddened nose, often a sign of excess alcohol or of liver dysfunction. Around his eyes there were small, yellow fatty deposits, known as xanthelasma, suggesting raised cholesterol levels and indicating an increased risk of heart disease.

I took his pulse, which was a regular 78 but seemed to be straining, perhaps indicating that his heart was having to work harder than normal. His tongue was healthy but mildly enlarged, traditionally thought to reflect poor digestive function.

Taken together, these signs suggested to me that he was on a path that would lead to metabolic syndrome, a condition that includes raised blood cholesterol levels, insulin resistance, high blood pressure and fatty liver.

He was a high achiever, I thought, who despite his relaxed manner pushed himself hard in a competitive world and he was just at the age where high blood pressure could become a problem. I fed all this back to him, displaying a confidence that didn't quite match how I felt.

"You are overweight and are not getting enough exercise. You need to eat less, you have raised cholesterol levels, and in the long term are at risk of becoming diabetic. I suspect you have mild to moderately high blood pressure, and your heart and your liver function need some support. I would guess that you drive yourself too hard and work too long hours, you are not getting enough good-quality sleep, and maybe drink too much alcohol (beer?). You need to exercise and relax regularly, and to continue with the diet recommended by your naturopath."

He laughed, and the Australian inflection in his voice became stronger.

"You've just about summed me up," he said. "I do get headaches but otherwise I think you've got everything covered. OK, where do we go from here?"

It was the start of a warm and enduring relationship. He came to see me two or three times a year to report back and monitor progress, and I looked forward to seeing him. We would talk over any health issues he'd had and I would encourage him to persevere with his diet and exercise regime, and to relax regularly. We enjoyed catching up and took time out to talk about the weather, his emotional state, life in Norwich or whatever was the subject of the day.

His blood pressure stabilised after a few months at about 130/85, slightly higher than hoped for but nonetheless acceptable. He lost 2kg but couldn't lose more despite keeping to a Mediterranean diet, and regular sessions in the gym before work. He had a regular annual blood test to check his blood, liver and cholesterol levels, all of which remained within or close to normal parameters. He didn't like taking tinctures and couldn't get round to taking them before meals, so I gave him capsules and tablets instead: artichoke, ashwagandha, ginkgo, olive leaf, turmeric and valerian being the ones routinely prescribed.

We worked together like this for just over five years, and it was a sad day when he explained that this would be his last appointment. He and his wife, Toni (who had also come to see me several times for herbal treatment), were off back to Australia. They had loved life here in Norfolk but home and family were calling. They would get back in touch with their naturopath in Melbourne—they greatly valued all that I had done for them.

I have the card they gave me, a woodland scene, their kind words within.

Not as they seem

Iwas just into my third year in practice, when a woman in her early twenties came to see me with itchy eczema on her arms and legs. She looked ill at ease in the waiting room, every so often rubbing or scratching along the length of her arms and behind her knees.

"Oh, I'm so glad to be seeing you," she said, as she sat down her chair. "I've seen ______ (a fellow herbal practitioner who worked nearby) for two months and there's been no improvement. I've been told you're much more skilful than her I know you can get me better!"

She sat back, looking at me—a fixed, brilliant smile on her face, having said her piece. Uhoh! I went within, as I struggled to take in what she'd just said.

I should have read the warning signs and challenged her head on about the put-down of my colleague. I should have rejected the false praise. Instead, I avoided confrontation and said that eczema was a difficult problem to resolve at the best of times and that there were no guarantees that I would do any better. As she would doubtless know, even if the skin healed, the eczema could always recur and flare again.

I carefully examined her skin and noted the tell-tale signs of chronic itching—dry, flaking skin and tracks of small scabs, where the nails had broken through. Her skin was very dry but otherwise fine. She suffered mild hay fever with tree pollen in the spring and her menstrual cycle was irregular and occasionally heavy. Her tongue indicated that she might be anaemic, her pulse was faster than expected.

After discussing a range of possible treatments with her, I recommended that she try applying neat evening primrose oil to itchy areas, and made up a tincture containing red clover, calendula, passiflora and Oregon grape. She left looking happy, clutching her new medication.

She came back two weeks later, having done well—her skin was much more comfortable and the itching had almost stopped, she was sleeping better and had more consistent energy. I suggested adding chaste berry to her tincture, as this could help regulate her menstrual cycle. She agreed, and I made her up enough tincture to last till her next appointment in four weeks' time.

Two weeks later, she left a message while I was at lunch, asking me to call back urgently. When I got back to the clinic and called her, she told me in a terse voice that she was not doing well and needed to see me immediately. I explained that I was full up for the rest of the day—could she come and see me tomorrow? No, she had to be seen today. Reluctantly, I told her she could come at 5pm. I had a new patient booked in at 5pm, so would only be able to see her for a few minutes.

Just before 5pm I came down to reception and saw her sitting there, scratching furtively at her arms and legs, a gaunt look on her face. I went over to my 5 o'clock patient, explained that I would be with him in 5 minutes, and asked her to come through to the consulting room.

As I sat down, she turned on me and said, "You're trying to poison me."

The words were spat out and the shock I felt was almost physical. I was thrown as much by the vehemence with which she spoke, as by the wild accusation. She seemed a quite different person to the one I had seen before.

In that instant, I became aware that a large dark, threatening hole had just opened up and yawned before me. It would not be difficult to fall in and be trapped. Like it or not, I had arrived at a defining moment in my life as a herbalist. Should I fail to find a path around this false accusation, my future could be swallowed up for months, even years ahead. Despite being innocent, my practice would be examined and presuming 'no smoke without fire', my reputation damaged.

"I am very sorry that you feel this way," I said summoning up every fibre in my being, "but I can absolutely assure you that I am not poisoning you."

She sat there, fidgeting with her hair, staring at me almost as if half of her was not there, vacant, and the other half possessed by the Furies.

"I want *all* my money back, the appointments and the herbs."

The extreme tension in my body slackened a little and I breathed a sigh of relief. There *was* a way ahead. If she was after money, then that could be dealt with, though instinct told me that caving in too easily and returning all that she had paid would not be a good idea. It might be taken as weakness and a partial admission of guilt.

"You told me you did well with your first prescription, and you made no complaint at either appointment, so I can't give you the money back for these. But you are clearly unhappy with your last prescription and haven't done well with it, so I can give you back what you paid for this last prescription." I held my breath and prayed she would accept the offer.

As I watched, I could see the struggle playing out across her face, her eyes jerking from one side to the other. She looked fraught and uncomfortable—she wanted to reject my offer, to have all the money back but couldn't find a way to do it. Grudgingly, yes, thankfully, she would take the money.

I pulled out the notes and coins and gave them to her. She took them, avoiding my gaze, and without another word walked out the door. I sat back drained but knowing I had come through to the other side. After a couple of minutes, I went downstairs to see my next patient and to apologise for keeping him waiting so long.

A fair hearing

The front doorbell rang and I went to answer it. It was my 5 o'clock new patient. He was standing there, upright, almost with a military bearing, in his late seventies with snowy white hair, ruddy complexion and an expensive, well-tailored suit. He was taller than me and his blue-grey eyes gazed coldly down at me.

"Edward?" I said, eliciting the merest nod in reply. "Pleased to meet you, do come on in."

We walked into the consulting room and I sat down. Edward on the other hand remained standing, deliberately not sitting in the proffered chair. I wondered what was going on.

"My wife made the appointment for me, she's concerned about my health and wants me to see you. She has a lot of faith in herbal medicine," he said with a disparaging look. He paused, finding the right words:

"I am a retired High Court judge, and I want you to know that I drink a bottle of claret every lunchtime and that I am not going to stop doing this."

Hindsight is a fine thing. I should have replied:

"Edward, I know that in the High Court you are used to holding sway, but you are in my 'court' now. Please give me a fair hearing and benefit of doubt! We can discuss your health issues, and I will tell you what I think is best to recommend, that will be of most help. In the end, it is up to you whether you choose to follow these suggestions or not."

Of course, I didn't! I prevaricated. I said I would give him a diet sheet that would recommend the standard maximum of 15 units of alcohol a week, and that his current level of alcohol was clearly not advisable. No surprise then that the consultation had its awkward moments, and that he only came to see me the once.

In my experience, some of the most difficult patients to work with are ones, like Edward, who have been persuaded or bullied into making an appointment to see the *herbalist*! It can be a wife making an appointment for her husband (it probably does happen the other way around on occasion), parents for teenage sons or daughters, children for their elderly parents—the same problem occurs. They did not choose to consult you and, in their heart of hearts, may well not want to be there talking with you. You have to work hard just to get 'a fair hearing'.

This is a problem because 'hearing', unlike 'seeing', has to be a *mutual* endeavour. As a herbal practitioner, you are lost if your patient switches off and stops attending—hearing, listening, responding—to what you have to say.

Second time around, I was more prepared. Colin, a north Norfolk dairy and arable farmer, came to see me—sent by his wife, who was already a patient of mine. He was not a well man and had a long history of bronchitis and chest infections.

I asked him whether he got plenty of exercise and fresh air, being a farmer. He grinned mischievously and, with a typical Norfolk sense of humour, said that would be true, if I counted the ten hours he spent in the cab of his tractor each day, more at harvest time.

This didn't feel like an ideal start but I was determined to get him to listen to what I had to say. One of the best things he could do, I explained, to counter his recurrent chest infections, would be to take garlic at each main meal. He could crush a fresh clove and mix it into his food at lunch and dinner, or he could take capsules or tablets.

His expression made it clear that he would never, ever put garlic in his food, but more seriously, I could see that he was wavering and doubting that I would be able to help him—why was I faffing on about garlic?

There are over a thousand research papers on the medicinal benefits of garlic, I continued. It is a powerful and well-researched natural antibiotic. It may only be about one hundredth of the strength of penicillin but in the First World War, garlic was shipped by the tonne to the trenches in France and Belgium, because at that time it was the most effective treatment available for wounds. Mashed up and applied with sphagnum moss as a sterile dressing, it had a good chance of preventing sepsis and keeping battlefield wounds clean.

Later, I learnt that he had a keen interest in military history, but I had achieved my main objective—I had his full attention again.

In terms of your heath, and your tendency to bronchial infection, the key thing is that garlic's antibiotic constituents are eliminated from the body via the lungs—that's why people's breath smells of garlic, after eating it. These constituents support immune resistance and bacterial balance within the chest and airways, and help to prevent infection.

Unlike prescribed antibiotics, garlic has next to no side effects, can be taken long term, and has an impressive range of other health benefits—it's antiviral, counters fever, lowers raised blood pressure, lowers blood cholesterol levels, helps stabilise blood sugar levels and has a long-standing reputation in maintaining health, as one ages.

He looked thoughtful, and I could tell that he was listening, and had at last begun to see why I was talking so much about garlic. He was a practical man, so I thought I'd give him a simple experiment to try to reinforce what I'd just said.

The body is incredibly efficient, I explained. It starts to eliminate garlic via the lungs as soon as it enters the blood stream. You can try this at home: cut a clove of garlic in half and rub it on the sole of your foot. You'll smell garlic in your breath within about two seconds. He laughed and said he'd give it a go!

Colin had had bronchial problems for many years, and we were not going to suddenly reverse this situation. It was however realistic to expect that we could improve his overall resistance to infection, and reduce his need for prescribed antibiotics.

Along with garlic tablets, I gave him a tincture containing angelica root, echinacea root, elecampane and white horehound, and suggested that he drink regular cups of thyme tea with honey.

We got on well after this first appointment, and he continued intermittently with treatment for several years. His health clearly improved—Val, his wife, confirmed this—but when the weather turned each autumn he would again start wheezing and coughing up green mucus and need antibiotics.

He was of course a workaholic and never rested sufficiently. His family and his animals came first. We took to discussing how herbal medicine could be used to help his cattle, and he reported back positively, when the calendula and garlic ointment that I'd suggested proved successful in healing mastitis in one of his cows.

Eventually, I heard no more from him or his family. Had I been part of the local community rather than someone who had moved up from London, it might have been different. One of the hardest things in herbal practice is losing contact, and not knowing what has happened to a patient.

In the garden

Perhaps ten years later, in 1997, I went round one afternoon to visit Jane, a friend and fellow medical herbalist, who lived close by in Islington. We sat in her garden looking at the ceanothus and peonies in flower, deep blues and pinks scattered alongside raised beds filled with herbs such as sage, helichrysum and rosemary, and overshadowed at the end by several oak trees.

Over tea, we reminisced about herbalists we'd known who had retired or died, and how a whole new generation of practitioners was coming through, who for the first time were university-educated and had a thorough scientific training. They would bring an entirely different vision to the profession, we agreed, though whether they would have the same sense of vocation as previous generations, or an awareness of how much the practice of herbal medicine meant confronting the unknown, remained to be seen.

Jane started talking about Robin Nielsen, and I realised that she had met him several times. In the 1980s, she had taken her teenage son Brendan—who today would be recognised as 'being on the spectrum'—to see Robin for herbal treatment to help with his anxiety, anger and poor concentration.

Robin was balding, tall, thin and perceptive, and Brendan took an immediate liking to him. Robin took occasional notes but spent most of the time encouraging Brendan to talk about his life, how he slept, what he liked eating, what he experienced at school. Jane saw that Robin wasn't fishing for details, he was trying to gain Brendan's confidence and that he was succeeding.

Brendan began to relax and started to open up about his worries and the blocks he had about school and schoolwork. He didn't want to be a nerd and be a social outcast, but at the same time he thought most of his classmates were stupid. They didn't question anything, they didn't ask why they were alive, they just wanted to go to parties and drink or smoke too much.

Robin said that nothing was ever fixed. You had to keep alive to the possibility that change could happen in the most unexpected ways. No day was ever the same.

"I'm going to tell you what happened to me one day when I was 12," he said to Brendan. "It changed my life.

"My father was from Norway, and every summer we'd go and stay with my grandparents who lived in the far north, an hour's drive out from Tromso. It could hardly have been more different to my life in London. Both my parents loved the wilderness and we would spend days out hiking across the mountains and the moors, no matter what the weather, taking food and stopping by lakes and waterfalls.

"One morning we had been out for about an hour, traversing a valley, when we met an elderly Sami man dressed in a traditional red and blue coat. With rough-cut hair and a deeply creased, kind face he looked like he had literally just walked out of the mountains. My father and mother talked away with him—I could only pick up a bit of what they said.

"The Sami man was staring at me and gestured warmly towards me. My father explained that the man was a Sami shaman, a medicine man, and that he wants to give me something. He wants you to come back here tomorrow and stand behind that granite rock about 100 yards up the valley. He says something will happen that you will never forget. You don't have to do this, my father said, but I knew he wanted me to say 'yes'—I agreed straight away.

"At exactly 10am the next morning, I had to stand behind the rock further up the valley and, whatever happened, I had to stay there and not move. My mother and father would watch from up the side of the valley and would let me know when I could move again.

"All day I thought about what this might mean and what was going to happen. It took me ages to get to sleep. My mother woke me at 7am and we set off after breakfast. We arrived well before time and I stood behind the rock exactly as told, while my parents climbed up the steep, rocky side of the valley far above me.

"The minutes ticked by. I looked at my watch just before 10am and heard a distant rumbling sound like thunder. It came from over the head of the valley and was growing steadily stronger. As I stood there holding onto the rock, the earth began to shake, as if an army was on the march. Dust clouds began to rise in the dry air above the scarp and suddenly, the front runners of a vast herd of reindeer came pouring over the crest of the valley, galloping at full stretch, hundreds of them following on behind, antlers borne erect, and all heading straight down the slope of the valley towards me.

"As they drew closer, I wanted to turn and run, but I held onto the rock and watched in a state of fear and wonder, as the herd pounded towards me and parted—like a river in torrent—around the rock. Their huge muscular bodies went flying by, on and on, on each side. I could see the velvet on their antlers, the sweat and mud on their hides, and I managed to stand my ground and not to run. It was all over in a matter of a minute or two, and I stood there shaken but feeling as alive as I've ever felt."

Brendan had sat enthralled listening to the story and murmured, "If only something as amazing as that could happen to me." Robin looked at him and smiled, "I'm going to give you some herbs to help you to relax and concentrate but, if your parents agree, there's a challenge that might help you feel stronger and more confident in yourself and at school."

Brendan looked pleadingly at Jane, "Let's hear what Robin wants me to do, Mum."

"You must have felt uncomfortable being put in that position," I said, interrupting Jane's account of Brendan's consultation.

"I wasn't best pleased," she said, "but I gave him the benefit of the doubt."

Robin explained that he was going to prescribe a tincture that included lady's slipper orchid and vervain, that would be tonic and calming. It would help Brendan to be more focused and emotionally balanced.

"You're going to be 15 next month, aren't you, Brendan?" said Robin. "The day of your birthday, wake up while it's still dark, get dressed, have some breakfast and go out into your back garden, as the sun's coming up. Wrap up well so you don't get cold, and take a bottle of water with you. You should stay out there on your own in the garden until midday. Like me with the reindeer, there may be a time when you want to run, but stay out there—you'll be a different, stronger person when you come back into the house."

Brendan looked excited and disappointed at the same time. This wasn't the romantic adventure he'd hoped for.

Jane said she would have to discuss this with Mark, her husband, Brendan's father, but she thought they would agree to it.

"Mark thought it was fine," Jane said, "and couldn't see how anything untoward could happen in the back garden."

Brendan took his bitter-tasting herbs with enthusiasm and counted down the days until his birthday. Jane became increasingly worried, however, as she saw that he was growing obsessed about what would happen out in the garden on his birthday.

"We all got up well before dawn that morning," Jane continued, "and wished Brendan 'Happy Birthday'. He was buzzing, with an intense look in his eyes and couldn't sit still. Once he'd eaten, he got everything together, went out into the garden and sat fidgeting on the bench looking down the garden. The sky lightened and the trees shone out as the sun rose. He sat like that for nearly an hour and then began pacing up and down the garden, looking at the roofs and the skyline and then down at the shrubs and herbs.

"I realised then," Jane said, "watching him through the kitchen window, that this was no game. Brendan was getting ever more agitated, his expectations were sky high and his patience, limited at the best of times, was giving way to anger and frustration. He started gesticulating and waving his arms around, making low growling noises, until suddenly he let rip, roaring and raging away, cursing and swearing at everything and everyone, his face flushed and puckered with anger, so that I barely recognised him.

"It was a terrifying moment, his roars were echoing off the walls of the surrounding houses, he appeared to be absolutely out of control. I had no idea what to do and stood there frozen to the spot. I don't know exactly when it began to change but he grew calmer and slumped onto the garden bench, his head hanging down on his chest.

"I opened the kitchen door and told him it was fine for him to come in now. He looked up at me and said, "No, Mum, I'm not coming in,

I'm going to do this till 12, however hard it is." There was a certainty to his voice that was new, I'd got so used to his undertone of whining and complaint. I went back into the kitchen and found that last hour more difficult to endure than Brendan.

"He came in at last, looking ashen and completely exhausted. He mumbled to me and went over to the counter and made himself a cheese and pickle sandwich. 'What's for lunch, Mum?' he said, his mouth three-quarters full, as he munched the sandwich. Topped up with food, he opened up. 'I don't know what happened out there, Mum, but something got released in all that screaming, I don't feel cross any more. Do you think Robin knew that this was going to happen?'"

Jane paused, and we sat there in the garden in silence, the ceanothus, peonies and herbs bathed in the afternoon sunlight, as we sipped our tea.

The Garden of Eden

An old man, a donkey driver, appears in several stories within the Zohar. His aged appearance and humble occupation mean that he is frequently overlooked or dismissed by those around him. In one story, two Rabbis meet one evening in Tyre. After a long day's travelling, Rabbi Yose expresses his delight at meeting a fellow Rabbi, whose face shows signs of great holiness and learning. All day on the road, he complains, he has been pestered by an old donkey driver, who spoke to him only in riddles. They were empty words and, as they journeyed, he became increasingly more annoyed at the man's foolishness.

The donkey driver was close by at the time and they called to him. He came over and spoke to them, again in riddles, apparently empty words. Quickly, however, the pair realise that what they are hearing is the reverse of empty words — the donkey driver has taken on a humble guise and his riddles are words of profound, radiant wisdom.

Astonished, they throw themselves on the ground before him and listen in awe as he reveals hidden insights from within the Torah.

* * *

We met at Linda's house, a small terraced cottage in Harringay that backed on to the park. We sat chatting in her living room looking out through the French windows to a tiny courtyard garden, crammed with herbs and plants in pots. Denise had said she might be late, so we introduced ourselves and talked about what we hoped to get out of the day.

There were six of us. I knew Matthew, an osteopath I often referred patients to, and Inez, who was a healer and Shiatsu practitioner, but not the other three. Sonia was a music teacher and clearly very sensitive; Raj, dressed flamboyantly, was an astrologer and fashion designer; and Linda, who taught Biological Sciences at UCL, had organised the day with Denise.

Denise had been a friend for about five years, so I wasn't surprised when she arrived half an hour late, looking harassed and disorganised. I knew her well enough—she sometimes stayed with us in Stoke Newington, when she came to London—not to judge her by appearances, and beneath her frazzled exterior was a disciplined and acutely intelligent woman. She had taken a Masters in Psychology at Cambridge, played the violin professionally, worked in publishing, and over the last three years had restored a small medieval farmhouse in the south of Spain.

This year, Denise had spent six months with the Inga people in the Putumayo region in the south of Colombia, learning their language and lore, and in particular, their rituals and use of herbs in pregnancy and childbirth. She had been allowed to take part in ayahuasca ceremonies, and experienced shamans had guided her in communicating with plant spirits and in plant spirit medicine. This is what she was going to share with us today.

Plant spirit medicine seemed fine to me in the abstract. I was quite happy to recognise that plants had a non-material spiritual reality, but I was sceptical that people brought up within western culture were truly able to interpret what plants were seeking to communicate. I had the same problem with astrology (I wasn't going to share this with Raj!), that yes, the planets—like the moon—influenced life on our planet but I wasn't sure how you could be clear what that influence was.

I didn't think you could, but that was not Denise's way of seeing things. She was uncompromising. When she had presented her MSc thesis at Cambridge, the assembled academics and professors had praised her work and intended to pass it with Distinction, on the proviso that she remove all reference to the 'spiritual' from the text. She refused, they parted ways and she never did get the MSc.

She started by talking about her time with the Inga people in Putumayo, how generous they were towards her and how deeply grounded and connected they were with the beings, the flora and fauna, around them. If you opened up your heart, she explained, and stopped your mind from pre-determined thinking, you could begin to sense the plants' presence, to hear them, to travel with them.

She took us through two exercises that aimed to develop this type of mindfulness. During the second practice, a phrase from a seminar I'd attended many years before came back to me: "The god in the plant is always happy."

Denise turned to talking about the plants themselves. Mugwort was the *Queen* in plant spirit medicine, and you needed to connect first with her to enter this world and travel to those plants that could bring spiritual and emotional healing.

Inez commented that it was surprising that mugwort was the Queen—a wayside plant, inconspicuous, almost drab, so easy to walk past her without ever noticing. It was true, I said, mugwort was a humble plant, with small grey-green flowers, the very opposite of showy. Linda pointed out that its botanical name was *Artemisia vulgaris*, named after Artemis, the Greek goddess of wilderness, nature and childbirth.

We carried on discussing the many plants used in herbal medicine that also featured in plant spirit medicine, most of the time their medicinal uses dovetailing.

After lunch, Denise suggested that we all go round to the nearby park, and see if we could meditate on, connect and travel with some of the wild plants that grew in a large semi-wild area, set amongst oak and willow trees. It was a sunny afternoon and not too hot, we should be fine for an hour or so. There were lots of plants to choose from growing in untended areas—burdock, shepherd's purse, comfrey, foxglove, yellow dock. We spread out across the park, and eventually I found a raised area with common mallow and yarrow growing close to each other.

I probably tried too hard to start with, that old double blind of "I'll try not to try" that makes it so hard to disengage one's mind, when you're trying to feel rather than think! It was warm and pleasant sitting there, and I started to look closely at the mallow, its mauve/pink flowers covering the plant in profusion. At first glance, the flowers appeared to have five petals, but looking more closely I saw that each flower was shaped as a single trumpet, each petal sculpted out from the trumpet and etched across in a deeper mauve. Every flower conformed in most details and yet bore its own unique patterning.

I was beginning to 'lose' myself in the plant, and to let go of awareness of my surroundings, when out of the corner of my eye I saw an elderly West Indian man walking with a stick, slowly, perhaps painfully, towards me along the path. I tried to ignore him and, annoyed, wanted him to walk by and leave me in peace and alone.

He came closer, in shuffling small steps, finally stopping beside me. I pretended not to see him but he spoke quietly to me. "You look so happy!," he said, dark, doleful eyes looking calmly at me.

"I'm looking at the plants," I said, taking a breath in.

"Yes," he said, "isn't it wonderful to be back in the Garden of Eden, and at one with the plants again?"

I looked at him, amazed, as if I had just been brushed by an angel's wing. He smiled and turned back to the path, and I watched as he shuffled step by slow step away.

Broken heart syndrome

I first met Ailsa at the clinic, when I began practising in Norwich. The consulting room where I worked had a calm, healing feel to it, upright timber and plaster in the walls, rugged oak beams across the ceiling. From the gabled window, you looked out to the half-timbered medieval houses that lined the other side of the narrow street. It was a sharp contrast to where I worked in London.

Ailsa was an acupuncturist and we frequently referred patients to each other. She was from the west of Scotland and had come to Norwich in her twenties to read English at UEA. She'd stayed on and married and had a son. She'd taught ESL students for many years, then retrained as an acupuncturist. She was skilful in her work and dogged in pursuing disturbances that lay behind a patient's ill health—I valued the insights she shared with me.

There was something typically Scottish about her, slender, dark-haired and blue-eyed with a wiry, terrier-like energy that, for reasons I can't explain, always made me think of heather and the mountains.

When Ailsa's partner Colin retired, they bought a fisherman's cottage in Blakeney, not far from where we lived in Langham, and rented out their small, terraced house close to the university, where Colin had taught Earth Sciences. We invited them over for lunch one Sunday and met Colin for the first time, although they had been together for over three years.

From an old Norfolk family of solicitors and land agents, Colin was a true intellectual, full of knowledge and curiosity about the world—geology and the environment but politics, culture, and as we discovered, music, music perhaps above all else. Having gained a First from Cambridge, he'd gone to work in the Sahel as a geologist for 15 years. He played the violin, spoke fluent French and passable Arabic, and was entirely Francophile.

He was about ten years older than me and I didn't immediately warm to him, finding myself thinking that once he'd put forward a view, he was unlikely to back down. He wasn't an easy person to get on with but as I got to know him, I saw that he valued intellectual honesty more than anything, and though often well hidden, had a deeply caring and compassionate side. It took a while, but eventually we became good friends.

We discovered that it was music that had brought Ailsa and Colin together, and it remained an important part of what kept them together as a couple. Ailsa played the flute and they would spend afternoons and evenings playing classical pieces, though with a glass or two of wine, they could be persuaded to play jigs, reels or airs.

Their other joint passion was birdwatching, and they would often leave the house at dawn and walk out towards Wells along the mudflats and tidal ravines, binoculars at hand to watch the migrating birds feeding at the sea edge, shrilling out and whirling away up in the sky, sometimes massed in their thousands.

Ailsa reduced her hours working in the clinic and in the summer months they would head off for weeks at a time to Scotland, staying with Ailsa's family in Edinburgh or Oban and then go north, sometimes as far as the Orkneys, finding B&Bs to stay in and mountains and wild terrain to explore.

One year they had been away for about two weeks, when I got an unexpected call from Colin one evening. "Hi Tom, I'm in Scotland at the moment," he said, "but coming back to Norfolk tomorrow—could I call round and see you sometime around five-ish?"

I didn't think anything of it and said, "Yes, of course, look forward to seeing you"—I had patients but only in the morning.

The next day at about 4.30pm, Colin's battered Peugeot pulled up outside the house. He struggled out of the car looking distracted and wild-eyed, some part of him not quite in control. I sat him down and gave him a cup of tea and was shocked to learn that he'd just driven all the way from Callander, dropping off Ailsa en route in Edinburgh, but otherwise without a stop. "Just over 8 hours, all told," he said. He calmed down a little as we spoke, becoming more coherent, but I could tell that something wasn't right.

"Yesterday, we went up Ben Vorlich. It's only 985 metres but it's my 34th Munro," he said, grinning like a boy. "It was a good long hike up to the top but on the way back down to Callander, I started to feel dizzy and lightheaded and had to concentrate on walking properly, Ailsa had to support me at times. I've been fine today after a good night's sleep but Ailsa gave me strict instructions that I had to come and see you, when I got back to Norfolk." He was clearly in overdrive, and I was sure Ailsa had expected him to break his journey overnight on the way back.

We went into my dispensary where I took his pulse and blood pressure and listened to his heart. There was nothing conclusive but I wasn't happy—his blood pressure was high and his heart and pulse were beating fast and irregularly, with signs of arrhythmia. If he didn't slow down he could have a heart attack or stroke.

I told him he had to make a conscious effort to relax—regular deep breathing exercises for 5 minutes at a time would be good, helping him to unwind and lower his blood pressure. He was in a hyper state and needed to break out of it.

I brewed up an infusion of limeflowers that he drank there and then, and dispensed a simple prescription of hawthorn, passion flower and valerian tinctures. He should take a teaspoonful four or five times a day. I didn't want to give him anything more complicated that might possibly interact with drugs he could be prescribed.

I thought about telling him to go to A & E but he was not actively ill, and I knew that he would accuse me of being overcautious, so I told him to see his GP as soon as possible, who would hopefully make an urgent referral. By the time he left he was more relaxed and his blood pressure had come down to a more reasonable level.

The first appointment he could get was in three days' time. The day before the appointment, Colin had a minor stroke and was admitted to hospital. I learnt about this some days later from Ailsa, who had caught the first train back to Norfolk and gone straight to the hospital. Colin was in a stable state and was making sense, but he was still in shock, his speech slurred and his left leg mildly paralysed.

There was hope that he could make a good recovery but this would depend on the quality of the rehabilitation offered by the hospital and on Colin's will power and determination. Ailsa took all this more or less in her stride and visited Colin every day, staying with friends who lived close to the hospital. I didn't see her for a week or so and only discovered fully what had happened, when I went to visit Colin in hospital.

Shortly after being admitted, Colin had been diagnosed with carotid artery stenosis, a narrowing of the arteries that supply the brain. Although prescribed a cocktail of different drugs, his blood pressure stubbornly refused to come down and he remained at risk of a further stroke. The consultant wanted to operate to widen his carotid arteries. Despite Ailsa's reservations, Colin opted to go ahead.

At first, the operation seemed successful but soon afterwards Colin began to get severe migraines and seemed more confused. When I saw him on the ward in bed, he looked as if he had shrunk, his face drawn and slightly lopsided. He tried to be positive and we chatted away, avoiding all reference to his situation, talking about trivial things, though I wasn't sure that he was really following the gist of our conversation.

After ten days on the ward, the hospital staff were keen to free up his bed. Ailsa argued as vehemently as she could that Colin was not well enough to go home and needed ongoing hospital care, but she was ignored and directed to get ready to take him home. She ordered a taxi but as Colin was getting up he had another severe migraine and started shaking, becoming mildly incoherent. Ailsa told the nursing staff that it looked like he was having another stroke, but they took no notice and she was forced to push him in the wheelchair to the waiting taxi.

They had hardly been on the road for 5 minutes when Colin had a second stroke, his eyes rolling up and his left side going into spasm. Ailsa was terrified and screamed at the taxi driver to turn round and go back to the hospital. Colin was rushed off for emergency treatment but when he came round back on the ward, he couldn't speak and was paralysed in both legs.

Ailsa told me all this on the phone the following morning, seeking my advice. Exhausted and overwhelmed by anguish and anger, she couldn't cope any more, couldn't see what she should do. I didn't know what to say but listened patiently as she poured out her heart—she wanted Colin out of the hospital as soon as possible and was going to find a nursing home that would provide rehabilitative treatment for him; she didn't know how she was going to do this, or how to pay for it, but she was going to do it; she was going to talk to a firm of solicitors who specialised in medical negligence; she was going to see her MP. Everything was falling to bits, Colin's life, her life, everything.

Over the next month, Ailsa fought on a daily basis to get some semblance of order back into their lives. After a week's temporary stay in a nursing home specialising in dementia care, Colin moved into a bright and cheerful room in a nursing home in Sheringham, close to the seafront. He was speaking again, though difficult to understand at times. It was clear though that he would always be wheelchair-bound.

The local council declined to contribute to the nursing care costs and Ailsa had no choice but to give notice to the tenants in their house in Norwich and put it on the market. She saw the solicitor and started a medical negligence claim against the hospital. She went too to see her MP, who proved sympathetic, and promised to write to the Medical Director of the hospital.

In amongst all this, she managed to visit Colin almost every day, taking the Coastal Hopper bus each morning from Blakeney to Sheringham. On warm days, she'd push Colin in the wheelchair to the seafront and they would sit and talk and watch the sea and the children playing on the beach. Later, she'd push him back up the hill to the nursing home, her body straining with the effort.

I picked Ailsa up from Blakeney one evening and brought her back for supper with us. She looked haggard and the blithe self-assurance that was normally there was missing. Her face was pale, her cheeks flushed, and she had lost weight, more than was good for her.

Sitting round the table, she told us the good news first. Colin was doing well adapting to life in the nursing home. He was reading again and she was taking in an endless variety of books for him to read—current affairs, Gaelic poetry, a history of the Soviet Union. He was listening to lots of music, and letting himself watch television, something entirely new. Ailsa said that she'd feared he'd get depressed and withdraw from the humdrum life of the nursing home, but no, Colin was joking with the staff, staying upbeat and learning to play the violin again.

The bad news was perhaps predictable. The hospital rejected any suggestion of negligence on its part and would contest any claim against it. Her MP and her solicitor had both explained that legal action would take years to reach a conclusion and that despite the strength of the case there was no guarantee of success. If they lost, they would be liable to pay the hospital's legal fees.

It was a bitter decision for Ailsa to have to make but she knew she didn't want to fight for three to five years and, even then, not be sure of winning. What energy she had, she wanted to use to help Colin be as well as he could be. The problem was the nursing home fees. Colin's pension would pay for about one third, but she would have to find the rest from their limited savings and the proceeds from the house sale. Another struggle had opened up for her, as the tenants were refusing to move and the estate agents advised that potential purchasers of the house had been refused entry.

Colin slowly improved. I used to go and visit him for an hour or so several times a month. We'd talk about politics, my herbal practice, books he was reading, or listen to music or watch a film. He lacked the proficiency that he had in the past but he was playing the violin again, on his own and once a week with a musician friend, who played the viola.

While Colin was doing as well as could be hoped, Ailsa was getting more and more depleted, her outlook and mood increasingly bleak and despondent. I prescribed a sleep mix for her—she was lying awake for long periods at night, and she had regular massage and acupuncture from other friends. Josie and I thought she needed time away to recoup and relax, and to have a chance to come to terms with all the conflicting demands and emotions at play in her life.

An old friend finally persuaded her to go and stay with her aunt in Edinburgh for a week, and she came back brighter and stronger, though it didn't last for long. She quickly tired again and was forced to confront the fact that if she didn't pace herself, she would get ill. Feeling guilty, she cut back her visits to Colin to four days a week, resting up and going for walks by the sea when she could.

Colin reacted badly to this, interpreting it as rejection, and for the first time staff in the nursing home complained about his language and behaviour. On top of this, there was pressure from the nursing home to catch up on missing monthly payments.

Ailsa knew she had to look after herself and went to see a nutritionist for advice, who put her on an exclusion diet. I was concerned, as the last thing Ailsa needed was a diet that might lead to further weight loss. Her diet was good, I thought, but she needed to eat more and to put on weight, to increase intake rather than take it away.

Suddenly there was Covid, the world was turned upside down, and visiting Colin and the nursing home became an impossibility.

Even Ailsa didn't get to see him for close on six months. Ailsa fretted and worried and they had long Zoom conversations, but it wasn't the same, and she could see Colin withdrawing into himself and becoming more emotionally distant. Later, she confided in me that this hurt more than anything—she felt lonely and helpless, exposed to the ruthless depredations of lockdown.

Early one morning, Ailsa phoned. I hardly recognised her, her voice was so weak. "Tom, I'm so sorry to trouble you, I'm feeling very unwell, I think I may be having a heart attack. I know there's all these Covid regulations but can you come and see me?"

I dropped everything, ran to collect my case, gathered together some tinctures and dispensing equipment, and left for Blakeney. There was no one on the road and the harbour car park was eerily deserted. The door to the cottage was on the latch and I let myself in. Ailsa was sitting there in the kitchen, gazing unsteadily at me, looking very frail, her breathing shallow and lifeless. Her cheeks were flushed an unhealthy pink, her face wan and empty of emotion.

"Would you be better lying down?" I asked.

"No, I think I'll stay here, I don't think I can move, I get dizzy and short of breath if I stand up," she said.

"There's little point in calling an ambulance but I could drive you to A &E," I offered.

She raised herself a little and said quietly, "I am *not* going to that hospital, and the last thing I need is to catch Covid there. Can you treat me?"

I took her pulse, which was fast, light and thready, but mostly regular. Her tongue was good, but her conjunctiva—the linings of her eyes— were very pale. She might be very anaemic. Her heart was regular but beating at over 100 beats to the minute—much too fast for someone at rest. Her blood pressure was 90/65. It was plausible that she had heart failure and she clearly thought that she was dying, but I had too little experience in treating acute cardio-vascular illness to be certain one way or another, and in any case I lacked the diagnostic equipment.

I told her she had tachycardia—a worryingly fast heart rate—and that this had several potential causes, amongst them acute stress, severe anaemia and heart failure. I remembered reading of the longstanding use of hawthorn together with chilli for acute heart conditions, and made up a small dropper bottle of the two tinctures. I told her to take 20 drops under her tongue every 5 minutes. If the tincture was too spicy and hot, she should sip some water but try and keep the tincture in her mouth, so that it was absorbed directly into the blood stream.

I explained quietly that hawthorn was well researched and used as a treatment for congestive cardiac failure in hospitals in Germany. It was an exceptionally safe remedy. The chilli gave more force to the treatment and stimulated heart function.

In the short time I had been there, especially with the effort of concentrating and speaking, Ailsa had grown weaker, and I prayed that this combination would have immediate effect.

There was no change at first but 15 minutes into the treatment and her breathing and pulse rate had both improved a little. After half an hour, there was no doubt that she was stronger—it was hard to pin down but it was as if, as her heart strengthened, so her consciousness was able to settle back into her body. She had been apathetic, silent, almost frozen, but now I saw a change—perhaps she had begun to realise that she wasn't going to die.

I considered how to build on this short-term gain, and produce a more durable, restorative effect. I made up another tincture with hawthorn, Chinese sage, angelica root, motherwort, liquorice and lily of the valley, and told her to take half a teaspoon with water every hour.

After about an hour, Ailsa smiled weakly and said that she would like a hot drink. Her hands and feet were warmer and there was some colour back in her face. Her pulse had come down to about 80 beats a minute.

"I wish you'd videoed me," she said. "I really thought I was dying. The change in how I feel feels almost miraculous. I knew herbs could be potent but I never thought they could work like this."

As she slowly strengthened, we talked quietly, and I suggested that I phone Alex, her son, and tell him what had happened. Perhaps he could phone her doctor, make an appointment for her and explain the situation and, on the day, drive her to the surgery. She agreed and as I was leaving, she thanked me and tried to crack a joke—a promising sign, I thought.

I told her to call me at any time and that I would be back the next day.

She was in bed in the living room with warmth still coming from the wood-burning stove. Alex had called the doctor and then rushed over, moved a bed downstairs, made up the fire, tucked her in, and made her a flask of vegetable soup. I went out the back to get logs and stoke up the fire and then sat down and had a good look at her.

She looked even more exhausted than before, but this was a pattern I understood. The acute distress that had gripped her yesterday had gone, leaving in its stead profound nervous and physical exhaustion. She needed to rest and—that word that seems to have been excised from medical vocabulary—convalesce.

Alex took her to see her GP, who was excellent. He listened closely to what she had to say, examined her thoroughly and told her that she wasn't in any immediate danger. He referred her to the local cottage hospital for an ECG and said that he was happy to go with 'tachycardia' as a description of what was going on. She seemed to be doing well with the herbal medication, so she should continue with it, at least for the time being.

Over the following weeks, I visited Ailsa regularly and saw signs of slow improvement. She slept better, and the night sweats that had troubled her gradually eased. She had slept six hours at a stretch and woke refreshed, she told me with glee. The ECG had been inconclusive but showed some signs of heart damage. She was still weak and had to carefully ration the limited energy she had, though overall her stamina was better.

I kept her prescription more or less the same but, once I thought she had the reserves to cope with it, I recommended she take a high-quality Korean ginseng extract. She noticed the difference almost immediately, taking a small dose each morning and extra doses when she began to tire. It gave her the confidence to be able to go to the shops or for short walks, knowing that if she started to collapse with tiredness, she would be able to find the energy to get back home again.

At long last, the nursing home opened its doors to close relatives and Ailsa was able to visit Colin again. Colin looked pasty and had put on a lot of weight but he beamed with joy when Ailsa came into the room, and they hugged and held each other for a long time, words coming only later. Ailsa had recovered sufficiently that she started visiting Colin twice a week, for an hour at a time.

After nearly two months I was still trying to establish exactly what had happened to Ailsa. She hadn't had a heart attack and she didn't have congestive heart failure, though she had something that had similarities to both. I kept on searching the internet, reading research articles and papers on the physiology and diseases of the heart.

I'd never questioned whether the heart was a pump or not, but there were papers arguing that it would be impossible for an organ the size of the heart to maintain its function *as a pump* for the billions of beats involved in a normal human lifespan. At the time it seemed like medical heresy, but I discovered that the dispute about whether the heart was a pump, or alternatively, a vortex or dynamiser of the blood, had been going on for centuries—Leonardo da Vinci had proposed the presence of vortices in his drawings of the heart in 1513.

The structure of the ventricles and the spindly, web-like muscles within them, the trabeculae, lent themselves, it was claimed, to the idea of vortical activity. According to who you read, the thin, fibrous muscles of the trabeculae were either 'embryological remnants' or promoted vortical, twisting energy within the bloodstream.

I wasn't going to take sides—the truth was probably somewhere in the middle. I was struck, however, by the concept of the heart as a dynamic, energising organ. This seemed to correlate with its role as the electrical and emotional centre of the body much more accurately than the standard mechanical model of it, as a pump.

And then I found it—broken heart syndrome! I'd never heard of it before, but Japanese doctors identified the syndrome in 1990. Brought on by extreme stress, emotional loss or trauma, the condition mimicked a heart attack, but rather than being the consequence of blocked arteries, it resulted from muscle weakness within the heart, most likely caused by high levels of the stress hormone adrenaline (epinephrine) circulating within the blood. Broken heart syndrome was reversible over time and, though it could affect anyone, was particularly common in post-menopausal women.

I phoned Ailsa and told her what I'd just discovered—broken heart syndrome was a precise match with her symptoms and it was reversible. I was confident that with time she would make a full recovery. I thought she'd be overjoyed to hear this, but she was furious.

How could it be that the medical establishment had never talked about it, never ensured that the media discussed it and that the public was aware of it as a reality? Was it just ignored because it was mostly post-menopausal women who got it? Or maybe it was because the condition developed because of emotional factors—touchy-feely things rather than hard scientific *facts*, like blocked coronary arteries? If only she'd known this before—she'd had two months thinking that, despite the herbs, her heart was going to give out one day soon.

She was silent for a while and calmed down, and then began to laugh. "Thank you, Tom," she said. "Knowing that … has given me back my life."

Castle Acre Herb Walk

There were about twenty of us in all, out in the Norfolk country-side on a warm July Sunday. Some were still straggling behind, chatting in groups along the footpath or bending down and taking photos of the plants we had just come across; others kept abreast of me, anxious not to miss out or wanting to ask questions, and some were up ahead, anticipating where we would be going next.

We were walking through fields and woodland, and I was hopeful of finding some unusual plants to talk about. We'd seen common herbs such as dandelion, nettle, ground ivy, hops and yellow dock, but it's always good to find the unexpected. Mixing botany, folklore, traditional use and contemporary scientific research, I aimed to give a thumbnail sketch of each herb and its medicinal uses, along with tips for accurate identification and cautions where necessary.

All the world knows nettle with its sting, but I drummed it into everyone that, if you are going to harvest herbs from the wild, accurate identification is essential: pick the wrong plant and you could harm yourself.

We walked along the side of the field and came to a bank covered in St John's wort, its flowers shining a resplendent golden yellow in the sunlight. It was still at its peak and I picked a stem, held up the flowers and leaves for everyone to see and began to talk about the tiny red-black oil glands that were dotted randomly along the margins of the petals and upper leaves. I gave the stem to the nearest student to look at and pass on and explained that these tiny red-black dots contained key active constituents, notably hypericin, that were directly involved in the plant's antidepressant, antiviral and wound healing properties.

In traditional medicine, I continued, St John's wort was prized throughout Europe, both as a nerve restorative and for its ability to repair and heal wounds. In Spain, the herb had once been known as *Hierba Militar*, the military herb, due to its supposed unique ability to heal wounds from sharp instruments—notably swords and knives, though in more contemporary mode, surgical incisions too. Abrasions, bruises, cuts and small wounds could be treated at home with an oil made with the flowering tops of St John's Wort and olive oil. Once infused, this oil could be used on its own as a salve or combined with essential oils such as lavender.

A traditional French recipe recommends filling a clear glass jar with finely chopped flowers and leaves of St John's wort, and thoroughly covering them with olive oil, so that no air can get in. Seal the jar, label it and leave it in a warm, sunny position—a windowsill perhaps—for six weeks. After a week or so, the yellow-green olive oil turns a deep crimson, as the oily pigments in the petals and leaves slowly dissolve into the oil. After six weeks, strain out the oil, bottle, label it and keep at hand for home use.

Some people were looking glazed-eyed at all this, but others were scribbling frantically, while the more tech savvy simply recorded me on their phones. A woman asked if the oil was absorbed or just sat on the surface of the skin. I said I thought it mostly depended on where the oil was applied. If you put it on your palms or the soles of your feet, where there were lots of sweat glands, it would definitely be absorbed.

In fact, a famous 20th-century French herbalist, Maurice Mességué, whose patients included Charles de Gaulle and Winston Churchill, always treated his patients with herbal hand and foot baths—soaking for about 15 minutes, rarely prescribing herbs internally, as infusions or tinctures.

We carried on down the path and came to a marshy area at the end of the field, with water mint, a stand of yellow flag and a dense patch of hemlock water dropwort, its tall, upright, mottled green and red stems looming over the other plants.

Here, I explained, pointing at the dropwort, was an example of why one needed to be so careful when identifying a plant. Hemlock water dropwort was easily mistaken for other plants in the carrot family, especially similar-looking medicinal herbs such as angelica and lovage. Hemlock and hemlock water dropwort had in the past been used *externally* as lotions to treat conditions such as arthritis and rheumatism, but they were so toxic that they were rarely used today.

Hemlock was, of course, the herb that Socrates chose to swallow, when forced by the authorities to end his life, and one would probably die from ingesting even a very small amount. We all stared rather sombrely at the dropwort, and it was time to move on.

Further down the path we climbed over a style and entered old-established woodland. Suddenly we were in a cooler, greener world, with dappled shade and sunlight shafting in. We found ash and oak, rowan and birch, and discussed medicinal and folkloric uses. On the woodland floor, there was enchanter's nightshade, bugle and dog's mercury, and to my delight, butcher's broom.

Butcher's broom is a dark green, spiny shrub with tiny white star-like flowers, and then round scarlet berries, set oddly in the middle of what look like leaves: except, as the botanists have it, they are 'specialised stems' not leaves! Butcher's broom stems were traditionally used to make a rough, abrasive brush—thus the name—though the roots are the part used in medicine, making a first-rate treatment for varicose veins, often in combination with horse chestnut seeds (aka conkers!).

Just over the two-hour mark, we arrived back at the farmhouse car park where we had started. We gathered round and I made a final summing up, hoping that they had enjoyed the afternoon and found it informative. We had found and identified 26 native medicinal plants, and I hoped that if they planned to use herbal medicines in the future, they would feel more confident and safe in doing so. I was happy to stay on for a while and chat and answer any questions.

There were always questions about personal health problems at the end of a herb walk—could herbal medicine help psoriasis or chronic fatigue? How much ground ivy tincture should you take for sinus congestion? Could you use thyme tea to treat threadworms in children? Could I recommend a herbal practitioner for their son, daughter or parent, who lived in London or Cambridge or further afield?

Eventually, there was just one woman left who'd been waiting patiently to talk with me.

"I haven't got a question to ask," she said, cheerfully. "I thought you'd be interested to hear my dropwort experience!" I nodded with interest, and she began her story:

"After breakfast on a sunny morning three years ago, I put on my wellies, went out into the garden and decided that it was time to tackle the hemlock water dropwort. We have a large garden and at the bottom is a pond and boggy area. There's always been a clump of dropwort growing there, it is definitely a thug and grows so fast that it starts to take over.

"Without thinking about what I was doing, I marched down to the dropwort and started pulling away at the stems and roots with my bare hands. The stems are quite tough, it was warm work and I began to sweat.

"After about five minutes, I started to feel giddy and disorientated. I stopped pulling at the dropwort and realised I needed to get back to the house. Retracing my steps back up the garden I became more and more unsteady, as if I was hopelessly drunk, and didn't think I would make it back to the kitchen, where my husband was sitting reading the paper.

"I stumbled through the kitchen door and then collapsed on the floor in front of him. I was still just able to speak and told him what I'd been doing with the dropwort. We talked over what we could do and both agreed that there was no point in calling an ambulance—if I was going to die I would be gone before it arrived.

"I lay there on the floor, unable to move, my breathing growing more and more shallow, but oddly feeling almost serene and seeing a white shining light ahead of me, my consciousness coming and going. My husband took my pulse, and it was down to 30 beats a minute.

"I lay there for what seemed like a very long time. Slowly, I began to feel my arms and legs again, my breathing strengthened and I knew that I was going to survive. After about an hour I was able to sit up again and by the next morning I was back to normal."

She paused, reliving the moment.

"It's not something I would ever want to repeat but it was a strangely peaceful experience."

And then, returning to her day-to-day practical self, she said finally, "Of course, I've learnt my lesson … I wear gloves now!"

One day in twenty-fifteen

A new patient had failed to show up for their appointment, leaving me with an hour's gap until 4pm, when my next patient was due. I was sitting reading the news on my phone and absent-mindedly going over a conversation I'd had with a patient earlier in the day—she'd been feeling miserable and downhearted, appetite poor and sleep a lot more disturbed than usual.

"What do you do before you go to bed?" I'd asked.

"Oh, we watch *Newsnight* at 10.30pm and then go to bed."

"What about watching the news earlier in the evening?" I'd suggested, knowing how distressing the news could be.

"We usually watch the *Anglia News* at 6.30pm and *Channel 4 News* at 7.00pm, as well," she said, looking a bit sheepish.

Sitting there in a clinic room in north Norfolk, the morning sun streaming in through the window, I was momentarily thrown and struggled to find the right response. I got carried away.

"If we were in Holt in 1815, when the Battle of Waterloo was being fought, news wouldn't have reached us here in Norfolk for days, maybe even a week. People would have been out cheering and hoping that Napoleon had finally been beaten but even then, we wouldn't have known more than a few details. Isn't it better to have some distance from the news? Most of the time there is nothing that we can do to influence things. The media circus just moves on from one crisis to the next."

I could have expressed myself better but compulsively following the news is undoubtedly bad for your health. I looked down at the phone in my hand, and thought, here I am reading the news, when I should be going over patient notes or doing a stock check—I'm no more immune than anyone else. I was still thinking about what to do, when the phone rang.

"Hello Tom, this is Gerald Wilson here. It's a very long time since we last spoke, maybe 30 years—I wonder if you remember me?"

I recognised the voice immediately. We'd known each other in Manchester, while he was doing his doctorate in Economics and Development. We'd got along well even if we hadn't seen eye to eye in politics.

"I can see from your website that you've had a successful career—are you in Norfolk now?"

"Yes, you've caught me between patients."

We talked about my life as a herbalist and author, and about Josie and our children and grandchildren. It was good to talk with him though in the back of my mind I was going, why's he phoned? Does he need help? And I found myself remembering the last time we'd met and gone round for supper with him and Dilys.

He was in London for five days. I wondered if he was going to suggest meeting up. As we talked, the memory of that evening 30 years ago kept running through my mind … we'd eaten in the living room, in candlelight, books and more books on all four walls, a coal fire in the grate. It was a relaxed evening, but then Dilys mentioned the books that kept falling off the top shelf of the bookcase by the door—always the same place. She couldn't understand it, she'd found the books on the floor in the morning, at least three times.

I realised that I had been missing bits of Gerald's conversation and that we'd been talking about me for far too long.

"So, how about you, Gerald," I said, "how has life been for you?"

"Well, Dilys and I are still together and we are based in Toronto. I had a normal academic life until 2008, when *everything* went crazy. I'd written a book that predicted the 2008 crash and suggested new approaches to productivity and to maximising effective resource usage. The book became an international bestseller in the US and Europe, and overnight every multinational CEO around the world wanted to get hold of me to talk through their company's financial decision-making.

"It was mad! It's hard to believe but I've flown over a million miles around the world. Apparently, I've flown more miles than anyone else in history except for seven people. I had my own jet for a while, but it was too isolating and lonely, so I fly scheduled routes now. Thankfully, it's become a lot calmer, since everybody started Zooming.

"We don't have children, but we set up a global charity for children's education, which Dilys runs full time. We live in Toronto but we also have houses in London, New York, San Francisco and Sydney. At least, these days I get to spend most of my time in Canada."

I was speechless. Not in a million years would I have imagined Gerald having a life such as this, but I could tell from his voice that he wasn't boasting, this was how it was, and he was still adjusting to the way his world had been turned upside down.

"That is some story … it's good you've managed to get some life balance back," I said, rather lamely. I would have liked to carry on talking but it was getting close to 4pm and my next patient was downstairs.

"Gerald, it would be good to meet up some time, but I know I can't make it this week. When you're next in London give me a ring and perhaps we can meet up. Please give my best wishes to Dilys. I'm sorry but I've got to go, my next patient is due."

That evening Josie had a yoga class, so I ate on my own. I thought about Gerald's story. I wondered how he'd managed to cope with such an intensely pressured life, but he must have ridden the success more or less effortlessly, as if surfing the crest of a giant wave. It was hard to take in. Dilys must have gone through a lot of stress too.

Dilys's face came back to me, looking edgy and unsettled that evening, as she talked about the books on the floor. Josie is quite psychic, and she said she'd try and see if she could sense why the books were falling off the shelf. She closed her eyes and we waited, looking at the fire, shadows flickering across the room.

After a few minutes, she opened her eyes and said, "It's not clear but I can see lots of things on the floor, a bit chaotic, maybe bowls, and there's a cat—I think it might be a cat jumping up and trying to climb the wall and pulling off the books with its claws."

Dilys looked shocked. In a strained voice, she said, "Before we moved here, an old woman lived in the house, who took in stray cats. The estate agents told us that she'd died upstairs and hadn't been found until about a week later. The cats had all been stuck inside and died.

"The house was a total tip, so the estate agents gave us the option of cleaning up ourselves and getting the first month rent free. We had to spend three days clearing out and cleaning before we could move in. When we came into this room there was rubbish, and plates for feeding the cats, strewn all over the floor.

"It was grim," she said, shaking her head.

We were silent, taking in the implications of what Dilys had just said. I knew that Gerald and Dilys would not want to talk about ghosts, even the ghost of a cat; they were Marxists, and dialectical materialism by and large defined their view of the world—ghosts and spirits were delusional, religion was the opiate of the masses.

I was just about to change the subject and talk about our forthcoming move to Bangor, when Josie said, "You could leave the living room door open at night and put a saucer of milk down on the carpet. That might release the cat from being stuck in its painful cycle."

Gerald was tight-lipped but Dilys looked at Josie and said she would give it a try, though she didn't seem convinced.

We talked about our plans for the future and our move to a house with a garden, and left, promising to keep in touch. Just before we moved, Dilys rang and spoke with Josie. She'd done what she had suggested and so far it had worked—twelve days now, no books on the floor.

When Josie came back from yoga, I told her about my day and Gerald and his adventures. She laughed and agreed with me that she couldn't picture him as a financial whizz kid jetting from one executive boardroom meeting to the next, but then none of us had followed expected paths, had we? Who knew what the future held?

Peter

As we crawled along the two-lane road towards Amba's house, the heat was already shimmering, a mirage coming and going across the distant tarmac. We'd missed the Accra rush-hour but it was still slow going and we arrived a few minutes late to pick up Peter.

Kojo and Amba were all ready to set off for the funeral. Amba was dressed traditionally in reds, greens and yellows, Kojo had a bright yellow shirt—they didn't look at all funeral-like. Kojo had told us yesterday that his uncle was going to be buried in traditional Ghanaian style—in a silver and blue coffin shaped like a 1950s space rocket.

We would have loved to go too but Peter was waiting for us. He gave us a toothy grin, white teeth shining out against dark brown skin, and climbed into the back of the car. We turned round, gave Amba and Kojo a wave and set off for the hotel.

When Kojo had asked us if we'd look after Peter, we'd been happy to agree to take him for the day. Aged six, he was too young to go to his great uncle's funeral. What would be the best thing to do to keep him entertained, we asked? Neither Kojo nor Amba made any immediate suggestions, so we'd decided to go to a hotel with a large open-air swimming pool, where Peter should be happy splashing around for much of the day. All he needed was his swimming costume—could they put it in with his other things?

There was a pause, and then Amba explained that he didn't have a swimming costume. If I had been more on the ball, I'd have thought about this, but Josie told them not to worry, we'd buy some shorts for him to use before we picked him up. Later that day, when we went to buy the shorts, no one seemed to stock the right size and it was only after three stops that we found a navy-blue pair that would fit.

We parked in the hotel car park and paid at reception for a day pass to the pool and restaurant. We snaked our way through the lush, tropical gardens to the swimming pool. Peter and I went off to change and Josie relaxed on a sun lounger underneath the palm trees. Peter seemed quite happy to be with us and anxious to be on his best behaviour—having probably had strict instructions to this effect from his mum.

The trunks fitted fine, and we walked out over to the deep end of the pool, dazzled by the rippling sunlight. We stood there looking down into the water for a while and waving to Josie, and eventually I said to Peter, "Aren't you going to get in?"

He gave me an apprehensive smile, a tremor went through his body and he jumped, his sleek six-year-old body disappearing smoothly into the water.

Jumped was not the right word though, as he had simply taken a single step forward and then dropped feet first, like a stone, into the water, going way down and coming back to the surface with thrashing arms, spluttering and swallowing water, and showing signs of going down again and this time not coming back up—he was drowning.

Panic gripped me, as I realised he couldn't swim and probably had never been in a swimming pool before. I threw myself in beside him, lifting him choking and shivering onto the side of the pool.

Sitting there he took a few seconds to clear the water from his lungs and get his breath back, he looked a bit dazed but quickly recovered and seemed back to his cheerful, trusting self.

I cursed myself for putting him through such an ordeal, presuming that he could swim because he lived close to the beach! So that was why it had been so hard to find the swimming trunks—how many Ghanaian six-year-olds had ever been swimming?

Thankfully, there was a shallow children's pool. The water was very warm, and now laughing about what had just happened, Peter began to relax and enjoy himself. We tossed a beachball at each other for a while, trying to splash each other as much as possible, and when I could see that he'd settled down, I went and sat down in the shade with Josie.

After an about hour, we decided to order lunch and have it by the pool. A very overweight waitress wandered slowly out from the restaurant with the menus. Peter ordered pizza, Josie a salad, but there wasn't anything I wanted and I couldn't make up my mind.

"Well, what do you want then, Dad?" the waitress said, looking at me with that cheeky, wicked smile that Ghanaians are so good at, her body looming over me on the lounger, as she talked. So that's what she thinks, I thought to myself, sensing that this was not something she felt good about, and rapidly ordered a chicken burger.

She thinks we've adopted Peter, probably come all the way to Accra just to arrange it. Perhaps, there's a regular flow of childless white couples who stay here and adopt Ghanaian children, and that's what she sees in us?

I felt shocked and half-amused at the same time, eating the burger on auto-pilot when it came, my mind still fixed on cultural understandings … and misunderstandings! We all see what we expect to see, interpreting what is in front of us through the lens of past experience—it's difficult not to do it.

By about 3pm Peter was getting bored. It was time to take him back to his parents, who would be home by now. Peter and I waited in the lobby for Josie to arrive, and Peter, being the well-behaved child that he was, picked up the large bag with all our stuff for the day out, and then took Josie's small rucksack and put it over his shoulder, alongside his own.

We started walking down the long corridor towards Reception and the main entrance, Josie and I more or less hands free, Peter struggling to keep up with us, burdened as he was by the bag and rucksacks. As we drew closer to Reception, I noticed that the two people behind the counter were staring in our direction in a very attentive way. They were sizing us up and had pursed lips.

I couldn't understand why, until in a flash, I saw what they were seeing. Panic again! Here is a small black boy struggling with heavy bags and trying to keep up with a white couple who are striding along carrying nothing! They think we have off-loaded our bags onto our adopted black son, and following in the all too recent footsteps of colonial history are treating him as a servant or worse.

I grabbed the heavy bag from Peter without a word, held it against my chest with both hands, and putting a brave face on it, with Josie and Peter quite unawares, we sauntered past Reception and out of the hotel into the heat of the car park. We found the car, put the air conditioning on max and set off to take Peter back home.

Encounters

It was late June and the hedgerows were full of the scent of honeysuckle and wild thyme. Walking the byways and paths of Anglesey, *Ynys Mon* in Welsh, had made us fit and strong, striding out each day towards the coast or inland, the views across the Menai Straits to Gwynedd and the Snowdon mountain range halting us again and again in our tracks, a view so hauntingly beautiful, so changeable with cloud and tide, that it became etched deep in my mind. From Great Orme's Head to the Menai bridge, the mountains rise up and waver far across the horizon, sometimes grey, sometimes green, even purple with the heather in flower.

Yesterday, we'd walked up through Glan-yr-afon, a hamlet with few trees and strewn with granite boulders, giving it an authentic edge-of-wilderness feel. On up towards Mariandyrys, turning off the road and hiking over the gently curving top until the roar of the Irish Sea on the rocks below and a distant glimpse of the Isle of Man replaced the hedgerows and birdsong.

It was boggy going, boots sinking into the sphagnum moss well above our ankles, and then—the surprise!

There it was, in a sheltered spot a few metres back from the cliff face and surrounded by short grass—an exquisitely beautiful, ivory-white flower, green tracings across its five petals. From a rosette of heart-shaped leaves rooted in the damp humus and on an upright green stem, the solitary flower shone out like a star in the midst of the bog. Swaying occasionally, a honeyed scent carrying in the breeze, it seemed too delicate to be flourishing in so wild a place.

We were held captive, momentarily speechless, before it—knowing nothing about it or what it was.

Back home with a mug of tea and dry feet and socks, we leafed through the flora until we found it, quite unmistakeable—grass of Parnassus (*Parnassia palustris*). This, we agreed, had to be one of the most romantic names of any English wildflower, certainly a contrast with its common name, bogstar.

First listed nearly two thousand years ago in *Materia Medica*, a vast work on medicinal plants by Dioscorides (c. 70CE), the plant was described as having 'ivy-like leaves and a fragrant white flower'. Disappointed, we realised with such vague details there was no way of knowing what plant was being described—it might be our grass of Parnassus, it might not.

Josie had had enough, she had a meeting in Bangor the next morning and went to bed, but I carried on reading. It was fifteen hundred years until grass of Parnassus was accurately described, in *Stirpium adversaria nova* (New notes on plants 1570), an early scientific work on medicinal plants, dedicated to Queen Elizabeth I, by the Flemish physician and botanist, Matthias de l'Obel or Lobel (b. Lille, Flanders 1538, d. Highgate, London 1616). I had never heard of Lobel before, though his name lived on in the genus of flowering plants that bore his name—*Lobelia*.

When it came to medicinal use, there was little to be found. An infusion of the leaves was astringent, and the distilled water had been used as an eye lotion. Due to its heart-shaped leaves, it had once been considered a heart tonic. Poorly researched, one paper reported that it might have 'tumour cytotoxicity'.

At this point that was enough for me too. A new plant had arrived in my life—tomorrow, I would go back with my camera.

I was up early and, after a quick breakfast, was out on the road. It was a fine morning and I followed the same route, this time skirting the worst of the bog and keeping my feet dry. The light was good and with fresh eyes I marvelled again at the beauty of the flower, noting for the first time the single leaf on the stem and the yellow-gold stamens, set proud above the five petals.

There was little wind and I took lots of close-ups, as well as photos with the sea or cliffs as background, and once I was certain I had a good selection, I clambered back up towards the crest of the hill, knowing that the whole expanse of the island, the straits and the Snowdon mountains would be waiting for me at the top.

The air was clear, sailing dinghies were scudding across the bright, choppy water and I could make out a train hugging the north Wales coast, the mountains rising up behind it, fold on fold.

I stopped and drank it all in, and after a few minutes set off down a lane I'd not walked before, high hazel hedges and thick green turf along the centre. The lane twisted and turned, and round a sharp corner I encountered a man in worn tweeds and a cloth cap leaning on a farm gate.

"Bore da, good morning," I said,

"Good morning to you," he replied, "a fine morning, it is."

He had a gentle, windswept face, hair white and sharp, intelligent, sparkling grey eyes that belied the tremor in his hands, holding on the gate. I recognised the lilt in his voice, the same as my grandmother, who'd been born near Holyhead and spoke Welsh as a child.

He had a quiet dignity and was clearly pleased to have company. Life had not been easy—in the 1930s he'd left his parents' small farm here and gone to work in the slate quarries in Bethesda. Hard, gruelling work, it was. The conditions were terrible but there was little work to be had elsewhere. He was a Labour man and after a while he'd organised the union at the quarry.

They'd put in for better conditions, better pay, and gone on strike when their terms had been rejected out of hand. The strike lasted three weeks and when everyone went back—no increase in pay, no change to conditions—he'd been sacked, and blacklisted across the whole of north Wales. Unable to find anyone who would employ him, he'd had to come back to his parents' farm and take it over.

"I've lived here ever since, and my parents long gone," he said. "Aneurin Bevan was the man, Welsh and had the right ideas. Tony Benn's the man now, but I'm not sure he's got what it takes."

He asked me where I'd been and I showed him the photos on my camera and told him where we'd found the grass of Parnassus. "Ah, yes, it doesn't grow on the farm but I've found it often in boggy places over the years. It's *Glasswellt y Parnassus* in Welsh, more or less the same as the English."

We said goodbye and I walked on thinking about our conversation, and about the photos, a few stood out.

I was cooking lunch in our shared kitchen when our landlady, Mary Roberts, came in. "What have you been up to today?" she asked, so I showed her the photos and told her I'd met this farmer on the way back and had a long, interesting talk with him.

"Ah," she said, "that will be Gwylim Wyn Jones. I haven't seen him in a good long while, keeps himself to himself, you know, but he's well-known as a poet here, won the Chair at the Eisteddfod twice for his poetry. He's written some beautiful poems, in Welsh, of course."

Two thousand words

Here again, that too familiar feeling of being got at, of being strangely helpless, of being at the wrong end of authority. It's not clear if it's at school or work or home but loud and clear it's coming over: "You're not pulling your weight … lacking commitment … boorish behaviour … not being present … wasting our time."

The voices echo across the room, and like an unwanted end of term report, state that my delinquent behaviour has been noted, meetings have been convened. Voices whisper in my ear: "… sanctions may be applied … Pay attention, we are *talking* to *you*! … we are watching … sit up straight … benefits will be withdrawn … make our displeasure known to you forthwith … Come here this minute …"

I'm drowning in fog, I might be a dog, I rhyme to myself. I'm going under and you don't understand, I *am* misunderstood.

Slowly, I am breathing again, my chest moves, inflates and takes in air. I escape down concrete stairs and out from the building. I walk along a drab, grey canal path. It is cloudy and the canal stretches out unmoving, turbid, straight to the distance.

At last, as the dream evaporates, I wake with a pounding chest, a heart filled with angst. As consciousness returns, so does the memory of that injustice all those years ago. The anger still simmers there beneath the surface, like some quiescent forest fire that burns unseen within the subsoil. So many years ago, and here I am quivering. It seems far-away but it's there, buried within.

* * *

He's 13 or 14, this boy. Waiting at the bus stop across the road from his school. He can see the chemistry labs on the first floor, the lab assistant is clearing up. Early autumn leaves swirl along the pavement, a light breeze pushing them here and there. No rain.

He's a good boy, this one, he's been well brought up. Not beyond a bit of mischief and dissembling, mind you, but good hearted and sensitive, the kind that blushes when someone else is accused of wrongdoing.

He has plenty of friends at school but no one he can really open up to, no one to share his problems with. His mother is exhausted looking after his younger brother and his father, well it's hard to say, he is a kind man but like many of the generation that fought in the war, much of the time he is far away, emotionally distant, certainly not someone his teenage son can confide in.

He's at the bus stop with other boys from the school, all day boys. This is a boarding school and day boys are inferior beings, though whether this is because they avoid the rigour of seven days' a week schooling, or because their parents might find it difficult to pay the boarding fees, is not quite clear.

He's got his boater, his straw hat, in his hand—what well-to-do Englishmen used to wear at garden parties and when out boating, with coloured ribbons round the brim.

He's messing around the bus stop with the other boys, waiting for the bus home. They're trying to trip each other up. He's not paying attention.

He doesn't see the older boy crossing the road towards them. He looks 18, he might be a prefect, he's walking up to the boy with the boater in his hand, he's got a droll smile on his face.

"I can see you're from Smythe House," he says, looking at the chocolate, cerise and chocolate band for Smythe House that's wrapped around the crown of the boy's boater.

"What's your name?" He's wearing a prefect's tie, the boy knows what's coming.

"Bretland," the boy replies.

"You're not wearing your boater, you know the school rule—you wear your boater at all times outside school grounds, unless it's windy or raining. Report to me in the Prefects' Common Room tomorrow morning at break. My name is Spillar."

He gives Bretland a hard look, turns, and walks casually back across the road.

The other boys have melted away from the bus stop. They slowly come back, shaking their heads and silently commiserating with Bretland. The general opinion is that he'll get a 500-word essay—could be worse.

The bus arrives, they climb upstairs and sit down at the back, looking down through the grimy windows at the school, as the bus pulls away.

Bretland is reeling—I had my boater in my hand, all he had to do was tell me to put it on. Why couldn't he do that, it's not fair, it *was* a bit windy. His heart is pumping hard, pressure in the temples, stomach taut, neck tensed. He's learning the hard way how to cope with injustice and being got at.

Off the bus and down the lane to his house, he starts to unwind. The smell and colour of autumn leaves, the watery, almost horizontal sunlight seeping through the trees calm him and his furious pacing.

His mother has supper on the table, it's a relief to be back home and around his family with their shared, unspoken warmth for each other. His brother is throwing food onto the floor, his father is talking to his sister about her artwork, his mother asks how his day was.

"Fine," he says, "I played squash this afternoon with Patrick." He's not thinking about tomorrow and going to the Prefects' Common Room—he's got too much homework to do anyway.

Upstairs he switches on his transistor radio and *Sounds of Silence* by Simon & Garfunkel washes over him. Sitting at his desk he looks out at the lights spread out in the valley below. Despite the clouded sky, there's something in the twinkling lights and darkness that is soothing, which lends perspective to his fears and insecurities. He settles down to his homework.

Breaktime finds Bretland knocking on the Common Room door. Spillar is talking with a group of other prefects, and he has to wait standing by the door, until finally Spillar walks over to him. "You know what the punishment is for. You are going to write a 2,000-word essay on Existentialism, and bring it to me by the 15th October, that's 10 days' time. Leave it in my pigeon-hole over there."

He points at the lobby where the dark-varnished pigeon-holes hang on the wall and, having nothing more to say, turns back to resume his conversation.

Bretland can't believe what he's just heard. Two thousand words for not wearing his boater; two thousand words, that's going to take for ever. And existentialism—that's ridiculous, he doesn't even know what the word means. He knows another boy who had to write an essay on Cups and Saucers, but this is totally different, it's absurd.

To say he is feeling sorry for himself might be an understatement. Yesterday, he was angry but now he is simply deflated, he's fighting off desperation and the urge to cry. He just has time to walk across the gravel and get to his next class on time, but the sense of desperation does not go away.

Back home that night, he sits looking out at the darkening valley, a new moon arching in the sky. He gets out his encyclopaedia and looks up Existentialism. He tries to make sense of the few paragraphs that detail the main tenets of Existentialism and the notes at the bottom of the page, referring the reader to existential thinkers such as Nietzsche, Kierkegaard and Sartre.

It is not completely incomprehensible but there's a voice saying, "How can I know anything about this, I'm 14. This is not something a 14-year-old is going to be taught or learn about, there's only about 400 words to copy, I can't do this."

With the sudden conviction of a child, he knows that he's going to write this essay on Existence, not Existentialism—at least this is something that he can grasp and write sensibly about. After lots of crossings out, scuffed paper and ink leaking from the fountain pen, he has written two thousand words, much of it copied from the encyclopaedia, though some of it is his own thoughts.

He puts the essay in the pigeon-hole as instructed and walks off with a lighter step. What a waste of time that was!

"Your name's on the board to report to the Prefects' Common Room," a classmate tells him during morning break two days later. He can't understand why—he hasn't done anything wrong. He knocks fearfully on the door the next morning.

Spillar is there looking furious: "I told you to write on Existentialism not Existence—I'm not accepting this," he spits out.

"Bring a two-thousand-word essay on Existentialism to me by Thursday next week at the latest." Bretland can't believe what he's just heard but mumbles, can't find any words and turns away, fighting off the tears.

If he hadn't been brought up so dutifully, he might have thought about complaining to his housemaster that this was unfair and unjust, that he'd already been punished quite enough for a very minor infringement of the rules. But this was beyond him. He didn't know how to find the words and hadn't yet learnt how to set about engaging with or challenging authority.

He did not even realise—had no inkling whatsoever—that he had been set to write Spillar's essay on Existentialism for him. Spillar would copy out Bretland's essay overnight on Thursday, and then hand it to his teacher—as his work—by the deadline on Friday.

"You're working late on your homework," his mother says, as she looks into his bedroom. "I'm sure that's enough for one day—go to sleep now." Again, he couldn't find the words to tell her what was going on, they were somewhere in his chest or throat but they wouldn't come out.

The six volumes of the encyclopaedia were spread out across the desk, each open on a different page with paragraphs on different existential thinkers. This time there was no alternative. It still didn't make much sense but he could see that each thinker expressed quite distinct ideas about human existence and the meaning of life.

If he started with a general piece about Existentialism and the struggle to find meaning in life, he could copy out each of the entries for the major thinkers. But they were contradictory: Kierkegaard believed in God as his starting point, Nietzsche had announced that 'God was dead'. At least he could understand some of what they were trying to say but when it came to Heidegger, de Beauvoir, Sartre and Camus he could barely understand any of it.

It's hard to know how much of this reading and writing lodged in Bretland's mind. He had no intention of actually learning from what confronted him, his sole aim being to get the humiliation and hurt out of the way as quickly as possible, yet some of what he read and wrote seeped into his thinking and stayed there. His ability to write had been sharpened by the first essay on Existence and quite soon he found a rhythm as he copied from the encylopaedia and scratched away on the paper.

There was something almost glamorous about the ideas he was copying. They belonged to a world as far removed from the caring but conservative environment of his family as he could imagine. The second time round, he was almost careless about how he wrote, anger just beneath the surface. The thinking in this essay added up but the writing was sloppy, he wasn't going to worry about being grammatical. Spillar could go and f*** himself.

He put the essay in the pigeon-hole by the deadline, as instructed, but this time walked sullenly away. He could not have expressed how, but some part of him understood that his entire life had just changed. Authority was no longer to be automatically trusted, it could be unfair, take advantage of you, entrap.

Existential thought made little sense to him but ideas about the struggle of the individual in a hostile world and the need to find purpose and meaning in life had been planted and taken root in his consciousness. From now on he needed to be sharper and more self-reliant, he couldn't afford to remain the accepting, unquestioning child that he was.

Without realising it, he was parting with his childish faith and beginning to see that the world was cracked or fractured like a broken mirror—it was supposed to be in one piece, reflecting back a true, wholesome picture, but nothing was ever quite what it seemed, each shard sent back its own distorted image. It would take years until he reconnected with this simple faith and sensed the oneness within life again.

His parents could not understand what was happening to him. They tried to talk to him but got only monosyllables in reply. At school, his behaviour changed, he saw through the façade that the school presented, rebelled and lost interest in schoolwork. William Blake, Bob Dylan and Nietzsche fuelled his rebellion. He started writing poetry, his head full of half-formed emotions and ideas.

Only youth and nature were truly innocent … the world of innocence and kindness was being crushed by the brutal world of self-interest, power and profit … nothing much was sacred … one had to rise above the mundane world and find joy and affirmation.

There was nothing exceptional about this, he was following the well-trodden path of the outsider at variance with the world, who yet secretly yearned to be accepted and to belong.

The dream became a familiar refrain within his life, coming back to haunt him, especially when dispirited or low. The words, the voices and the landscape would vary but the intent and the feeling of being got at remained the same. At university, he studied Philosophy and valued the way this sharpened his mind, so that he could recognise and understand people's thinking.

He had thought, naively, that his studies would bring a deeper awareness of the purpose and meaning of life, but the reverse was true—the more he analysed and relied exclusively on thought, the further meaning retreated.

"Philosophy will clip an Angel's wings. ... Unweave a rainbow" (John Keats, *Lamia*) became his watchword, and though he wrote a dissertation on Camus' *The Rebel*, identifying strongly with the credo of "I rebel, therefore we are", he began to see that only when you brought thought and feeling together—mind *with* heart—and learnt to develop a sense of compassion for yourself and for others, could you hope to find a deeper meaning in life, a spiritual direction and sense of joy.

* * *

One day, waking distraught—sunlight shafting through the cracks between the curtains, my wife asleep beside me—I was carried back to this young self and his existential woes.

As I fought my way back from the depths of the dream and back to consciousness, memories of that time strewn around like flotsam, a voice whispered within that it was I—my 14-year-old self—who had written Spillar's essay on Existentialism *for him*. Two thousand words and Existentialism—of course! How was it that I had I never seen this before?

In that moment, I understood that those essays, written under duress, were *mine*, my writing and thoughts, however immature, and something of an achievement in a 14-year-old. I had gained profoundly in writing them, despite the pain and humiliation.

And now, in some inconceivable way, I could see that those two thousand had been a gift—they had opened up the world and set me on an unexpected, questing path, where words and their meaning counted far, far more than would have happened otherwise.

Over time, this sense of gratitude seeped into my consciousness like a cooling water. Slowly, I have learnt to be grateful and to understand that nothing assuages anger like gratitude.

The wall at the end of the veranda

"Look at this," Josie said, pointing to the wall at the end of the veranda. Peering past her shoulder, there was hardly anything to see.

"There," her finger hovering next to the wall, and yes, there was a small, inch-long lemon yellow something, stuck to the wall. Lemon yellow with spots of black and white and ridged more or less like a geodesic dome was this something. An unknown curiosity in the Colombian countryside. I went back to my coffee.

Josie put a photo on Facebook—It's a bug, It's a beetle, It's a chrysalis, I've seen one before but don't know what it is. Not a lot of help. We forgot about it, but occasionally walking past the wall it was there unmoving, maybe a little shrunken. Had it dried out, was it going to turn into anything?

It had been there unmoving for five weeks, when Roni, painting the outside of the house, finally got to the wall at the end of the veranda. What shall I do with this, he asked, pointing at the lemon yellow something. Paint round it?

"No scrape it off, it's in the way," was on the tip of my tongue but I said, "Leave it—we'll have a small patch as a memory if it ever hatches," came out.

The next morning Roni was painting the wall at the end of the veranda. "Quick, come and look," he said, and there was this small, crumpled, iridescent green butterfly, struggling into life, quite on its own, into the unknown.

It fell out of the cocoon onto the veranda and wobbled across the tiles. Slowly its legs gained strength and its wings opened—dusky black with a red tinge. It was walking in a straight line, but where to, how did it know what to eat, what to do?

It carried on and fell off into the long grass. What force was driving it on, would it survive, hidden from view, this little miracle?

ACKNOWLEDGMENTS

Many people, knowingly and unknowingly, helped me in writing these stories, my patients amongst them. Thank you to you all!

Maria Mercedes Uribe, my wife, has always been my best critic, invariably finding flaws and pointing out strengths, wherever they could be found. When my confidence flagged, Boruch Simons was always there to encourage me to continue on. Jonathan Ward, poet with a lifetime of experience in teaching creative writing, helped me focus on what I was really trying to do. Many people read my stories and gave me feedback, especially Kofi Busia, Kate Chevallier, Jill Davis, Monica Henao, Dinah John, Gabriel Mojay, Nitya, Anne Roy and Rosa Sauertaig.

Lastly, my heartfelt thanks to Aeon Books. How fortunate I am to have publishers who were willing to let me change The Herbal Apprentice, so that rather than being a student guide to herbal medicine it became this work of fiction.

Andrew Chevallier read Philosophy and Literature at Warwick University and later trained at the School of Herbal Medicine, qualifying and joining the National Institute of Medical Herbalists (NIMH) in 1987. He ran a busy herbal practice in London and Norfolk for close to forty years. He is a past President of the NIMH and taught herbal medicine for ten years at Middlesex University, where he was a Senior Lecturer in Herbal Medicine (P/T). He is probably best known for his books on herbal medicine, particularly his best-selling *Encyclopedia of Herbal Medicine* (DK, 1996, 2023) and *The Home Herbal* (DK, 2023). *The Herbal Apprentice and Other Stories* is his first published work of fiction.